D0510765

OXFORD MEDICAL PUBLICATIONS

Teamwork for Primary and
Shared Care

WITHDRAWN
FROM STOCK
QMUL LIBRARY

BARTS AND THE CLINICAL LIBRARY
SCHOOL OF MEDIC
WHITECHAPEL LIBRARY e returned on or before
.ie last date below

Book are to '

2 3 NOV 2000

5/11/04.

PRACTICAL GUIDES FOR GENERAL PRACTICE

Editorial Board

Michael Bull, GP Tutor, Oxford.
J. A. Muir Gray, Director of Health Policy and Public Health, Anglia, and Oxford Regional Health Authority.
Ann McPherson, General Practitioner, Oxford.
John Tasker, GP Tutor, North Oxfordshire.

Teamwork for Primary and Shared Care

A PRACTICAL WORKBOOK
Second Edition

Practical Guides for General Practice 17

PETER PRITCHARD

General Practitioner
Dorchester on Thames
Oxfordshire

JAMES PRITCHARD

Management Consultant
Oxford

Oxford   New York   Tokyo
OXFORD UNIVERSITY PRESS
1994

SBRLSMD

CLASS MARK	W84.6 PRI
CIRC TYPE	ORD
SUPPLIER	PCHIS 12105
READING LIST	
OLD ED CHECK	

Oxford University Press, Walton Street, Oxford OX2 6DP

Oxford   New York
Athens   Auckland   Bangkok   Bombay
Calcutta   Cape Town   Dar es Salaam   Delhi
Florence   Hong Kong   Istanbul   Karachi
Kuala Lumpur   Madras   Madrid   Melbourne
Mexico City   Nairobi   Paris   Singapore
Taipei   Tokyo   Toronto
and associated companies in
Berlin Ibadan

Oxford is a trade mark of Oxford University Press

Published in the United States
by Oxford University Press Inc., New York

© Peter Pritchard and James Pritchard, 1994

All rights reserved. No part of this publication may be
reproduced, stored in a retrieval system, or transmitted, in any
form or by any means, without prior permission in writing from Oxford
University Press. Within the UK, exceptions are allowed in respect of any
fair dealing for the purpose of research or private study, or criticism or
review, as permitted under the Copyright, Designs and Patents Act, 1988, or
in the case of reprographic reproduction in accordance with the terms of
licences issued by the Copyright Licensing Agency. Enquiries concerning
reproduction outside those terms and in other countries should be sent to
the Rights Department, Oxford University Press, at the address above.

This book is sold subject to the condition that it shall not, by way
of trade or otherwise, be lent, re-sold, hired out, or otherwise circulated
without the publisher's consent in any form of binding or cover
other than that in which it is published and without a similar condition
including this condition being imposed on the subsequent purchaser.

A catalogue record for this book is available from the British Library

Library of Congress Cataloging-in-Publication Data
Pritchard, Peter.
Teamwork for primary and shared care : a practical handbook /
Peter Pritchard, James Pritchard.—2nd ed.
(Practical guides for general practice ; 17)
Includes bibliographical references and index.
1. Health care teams.   I. Pritchard, James.   II. Title.   III. Series.
R729.5.H4P75   1994   610.69—dc20   94-17696
ISBN 0 19 262527 6 (Pbk)

Typeset by Latimer Trend & Company Ltd, Plymouth
Printed in Great Britain by
Biddles Ltd, Guildford and King's Lynn

Foreword to first edition

Dame Rosemary Rue, DBE

There must be numerous practices where attempts to acquire management skills have failed, or where the benefits of management courses have been lost due to the passage of time and changes in personnel. For those resolved to make a fresh start, or wanting to revise skills, this new workbook offers a method which can be applied immediately, using the practice's own resources and timetable. Almost no preparation is required: any practice that can book a meeting attended by all the team members can start at once. Busy primary care professionals are spared lengthy accounts of management theory, but should appreciate that the workbook is the outcome of many years of research and development in live practices.

The experience of the authors ensures that every word written is relevant and that the time recommended for discussion and homework will be well spent. Each week's work directly addresses ways of making the team, the very heart of modern practice, successful, efficient, and happy. Under the clear guidance given in this very accessible book, the essentials of team management can be approached with confidence and enthusiasm.

Note on second edition

Dame Rosemary Rue, DBE

The demand for an early second edition of the workbook shows, encouragingly, that primary health care teams are serious about developing their skills. The authors have taken the opportunity to emphasize shared care, perhaps the most important way of delivering modern medicine to patients, and have oriented the book for the equal benefit of specialist teams. Shared educational experience leads to shared understanding and if both primary and specialist teams undertake the practical programme set out in the book, they will be led to thoughtful and satisfying shared care.

The role of the facilitator, expanded upon in this edition, has been much appreciated by successful teams. The identification of a facilitator may be the first step that enterprising self-starters should take on the path to improvement in the quality of their working lives.

Preface

Primary health care in Britain, and many other European countries, is undergoing a number of fundamental changes. These include the increasing recognition of lifestyle and environmental factors as determinants of ill-health, the greater emphasis now placed on health promotion and prevention of illness, new contractual arrangements for general practitioners requiring greater accountability and value for money, and major advances in information technology. The WHO/UNICEF Alma-Ata declaration of 1978, reflected in the report on the Health of the Nation, has increased the trend towards a broader view of health and ill-health than that provided by the traditional medical model.

Specialist teams in hospital are developing closer links with primary care, often with the help of facilitators or specialist nurses. The workbook aims to help them also to develop effectiveness in their own team and to work in cooperation with primary care teams. Medical audit is now an increasing concern of professionals and health authorities and trusts, and its implementation requires teamwork and facilitation.

All these factors point towards the need for effective teamwork in primary care and specialist units, as well as communication between them. This workbook presents a programme of learning and practical exercises that can be undertaken within each team, preferably with the help of a facilitator. The plan is for all the professional members of the team to work on team development in 13 weekly sessions of about one hour, with some additional reading time and homework. This method has the advantage of being focused on the key issues and tasks facing each team, and taking the whole team one step nearer to the achievement of its goals. Talking about teamwork is not enough: it must be worked at if it is to be effective.

Oxford   P.M.M.P.
July 1994   J.R.P.

Acknowledgements

The authors wish to acknowledge the help they have had from a number of people who have worked in this field for many years. Particular thanks are due to Richard Beckhard and his colleagues who developed the practical groundwork for health team development, to Dame Rosemary Rue for her support of team development in the Oxford Region over ten years, to June Huntington and colleagues at the King's Fund College for ideas and stimulus, to John Horder (Chairman of the Centre for Advancement of Inter Professional Education) for suggesting this workbook, to Penny Astrop, Lorraine Pengilley, and Janet Bailey for organizing the field testing, and to the members of the teams who have undertaken the field testing. Wendy Mitchell and Mike Holden from Humberside Health have suggested changes to the practical exercises which we have adopted. Elaine Fullard and Janet Bailey of the National Facilitator Development Project have been unfailingly helpful. We also thank many colleagues and friends for commenting on the text, or supporting the project in other ways.

Professor Ronald Fry and colleagues have agreed to our using material from their original workbook. Tina Tietjen has agreed to our quoting from her *Unorganized manager.* Wendy Pritchard and her colleagues in the field of organization development have generously shared their expertise over several years. Enid Leonard and colleagues at the Oxford Regional Library, Margaret Hammond and colleagues at the Royal College of General Practitioners, and David Perrow and Lynn Winkworth at Templeton College Oxford have been helpful with access to the literature. Sue Flanders has faithfully processed the text. To all these people we are very grateful.

Contents

Introduction

General practitioners, specialists, nurses, and other health professionals do much of their work on their own with their patient
or client. But the coordinated activity that is today's health care
requires a number of different skills and can only function effectively in a team setting. Teamwork is the key to many of the
emerging priorities for health care such as health promotion and
prevention of illness, as well as care shared between teams in
hospital and the community, particularly in domains like diabetes,
cancer and palliative care, the care of the chronically ill and
elderly, mental illness, or maternity and child care.

Teamwork helps all those working in health care, both professional and lay, to achieve their objectives better and more
economically. But once people are involved in a team, the aims
and ideas of others have to be considered. The doctor, though
bearing a heavy responsibility for the outcome, cannot dictate to
other professionals who are themselves responsible for their own
work. A dovetailing of objectives is needed for the patient to get
the best possible service. An effective team will be flexible, and
able to adapt to new activities and challenges which are part of
the turbulent environment that we all experience now.

This workbook aims to help members of health care teams
to work together harmoniously and fruitfully, using their own
resources, with perhaps some outside help in order to get the
process started. Teams do not always function well without a
learning process such as described here. The workbook is set
out in 13 sections (including the introduction), each with a practical
exercise taking one hour. In addition there is some reading and
homework, often in the form of a questionnaire. The total time

1

commitment is about 16–20 hours. The authors believe that this investment of time and energy will pay off a hundredfold in the more effective use of team members' time and effort, and in avoiding the frustration and demoralization of faulty teamwork and shared care. In order to start, there must be an agreement to 'have a go' and commit time and effort to the project.

Though the professionals in health and social services may work closely together on shared tasks in a closely knit team, their management structures and the legal framework in which they operate are very different. Their values and beliefs may also be very different. For this reason, the emphasis of this practical workbook is on goals and tasks, on roles and procedures, rather than a deeper exploration of values and beliefs, critical as they are for motivation. In the context of the team, good working relationships need to be built up, even when some attitudes and beliefs are not shared, so long as the differences are understood and respected.

In relation to the model below (Fig. 1) which shows a hierarchy of levels on which we operate, the practical exercises in this workbook focus on capabilities, behaviour, and the environment in which the team operates. These lower levels of the model are more open to change, but a greater understanding of and respect for other team members' identity, values, and beliefs is essential in bringing about that change. The aim of the workbook is not to achieve total agreement between team members, but rather to encourage a productive working relationship, within which people can have the greatest possible freedom to work effectively, both together and as individuals.

Teamwork is a skill that can be learned, provided people are prepared to make the effort. Once learned, the benefit should be apparent—to patients in better care, to staff in greater job-satisfaction, and to the team as a whole in higher morale, a greater sense of achievement, and mutual support in the uncertainties and failures that are an integral part of all health care.

As illness related to lifestyle becomes a more prominent determinant of health, different approaches are needed to patients'

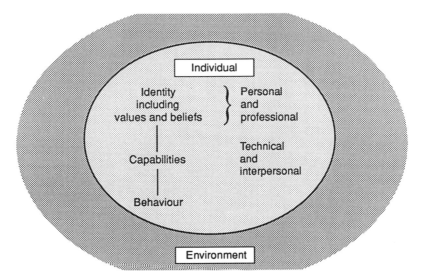

Fig. 1. Factors in team development—a model.

health beliefs and perceptions of risk. The traditional cooperation between doctors and community nurses has become more important with increasing day-surgery and early discharge from hospital. The newer profession of practice nurse has shown the most rapid expansion of all. The move of many patients from hospital to community care has emphasized the need to work closely with community psychiatric nurses and social workers. In all these areas, a team can only function effectively if the various members all work together for the patient's good.

For team-building to have any hope of success, all members must feel comfortable with the idea of working more closely and harmoniously together. One's own prejudices should be recognized and there must be a feeling that all team members value each other for the important contribution that each can make. In this way, the working relationships can be positive and open, in a spirit of equity, rather than allowing professional rivalries and 'pecking orders' to sour the atmosphere and run counter to good patient care.

Ways of using the workbook

For achievement of its aim, this workbook needs to be studied by all the participants in this team-building project, and the exercises in each section worked on in a series of about 13 meetings. In most cases this can be done in meetings lasting one hour, for example at lunch time. By working on team-building in your own place of work, real-life problems can be used as examples. Teamwork can be related to everyday problems and tasks. The orientation of this book is towards getting on with the job, but some reflection and homework will be needed too. If professional team members are prepared to invest their time and energy in this project, a clear message will go out that they are seriously committed to improving teamwork.

Ideally, the workbook should be taken as a whole by the whole professional team over a period of about three months. This may be a difficult option for some teams, and alternative methods can be considered. For example, in the case of Primary Health Care (PHC) teams, the partners and practice manager might work through it first, and then involve other professional staff in one project, and the lay staff and practice manager in a separate team-building project. Lay members of PHC teams, such as receptionists and secretaries, are equally important and their team-building needs should not go by default. In hospital, it may be difficult to decide who are 'core' team members, but a pilot project would soon identify who was needed to make team care effective.

General hints for conducting exercises

At least one hour will be needed for each exercise. This could be fitted into a lunchtime meeting if people arrive on time, and eat their sandwiches quietly. Some doctors may prefer evening meetings, but by having a meeting during (paid) working time, other professional and lay staff, will get the message that the doctors are equally committed to the success of the team-building project. For all sessions there will be some preliminary homework, for example reading a section of the workbook and completing a questionnaire or index cards.

In larger teams, it might be better to subdivide into 'firms' or other smaller groupings, in order to keep the teamsize small— preferably not more than ten (see p. 20 on size of teams). Small size can help overcome the considerable obstacles to interprofessional cooperation, by providing a safe setting. Sub-projects described in the practical exercises and summarized on p. 7, may well have different leaders, depending on the nature of the project.

The exercises described are only suggestions and guidelines. There is much to learn about the best way to approach team-building, and teams may prefer to develop their own exercises to suit their circumstances. However, without care it can be a minefield, and teams would do well to keep to the general pattern and ordering of topics in the workbook, as this has stood the test of time. Team members should be in the best possible frame of mind to be open with one another.

The role of the facilitator

The work you will do during the practical sessions of this pro-gramme concerns the way you work together as a team. As every team member is intimately involved, it may help to have a facilitator from outside the team to guide the process of the exercise. This person may be provided by the FHSA (or other authority) or an independent consultant. Their specific role will vary depending on the objectives of the session and the particular team but is likely to be one of managing boundaries. They will ensure the available time is used well and that the agreed ground rules are being respected (see introductory exercise). They may also summarize, reflect or interpret the processes the team are engaged in, in order to clarify issues of teamwork. Their position outside the team allows them to provide an objective view of these issues.

If no outside facilitator is available for some or all of the exercises, one team member will need to adopt this role. It is particularly difficult to be both inside and outside the team and so this 'in-team facilitator' must be clear which role (team member or facilitator) they are carrying out at any particular time. Other team members can help by understanding the difficulty of the dual role and treating the facilitator gently!

Each exercise has a summary for facilitators, which may help to ensure that the session runs smoothly.

Introductory learning exercise: Balancing the benefits of teamwork against the barriers to effective teamwork. Setting the ground rules for group working

Aims: To explore the benefits of, and barriers to, good team-working; and to set the ground rules for the exercise.

Objectives: By the end of the session participants will have:

(1) compared their views on the benefits and barriers to teamwork;
(2) discovered whether the benefits outweigh the snags;
(3) decided whether there are any barriers that need to be addressed;
(4) decided whether or not to use an outside facilitator for the remainder of the project;
(5) developed a clearer idea of what teamwork means to them;
(6) agreed to the ground rules for subsequent sessions.

Summary of practical work

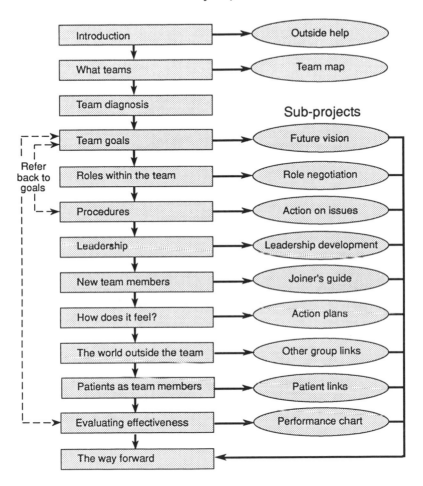

Fig. 2. The left-hand column lists the topics of the sections and practical exercises of the workbook. In the right-hand column are listed the sub-projects that may arise from the practical exercises, if the team decide that they would be useful, and time can be found for it. Sub-projects may not involve the whole team and may have different leaders.

Setting and equipment

Ideally, team members should be able to sit comfortably in a circle, so that they can all see each other, and no one has a position of dominance. Punctuality is important in order to achieve a productive hour. Freedom from telephone calls and other interruptions should be ensured, in so far as is possible. A good stock of index cards (about 6″ × 4″, 15 × 10 cm) will be needed. A flip-chart and marker pens or blackboard might be helpful. If no flip-chart is available, large sheets of thick paper stuck to the wall with 'blue tack' will suffice.

Exercise

Each team member should have a workbook and a supply of index cards. If necessary a few minutes should be allowed for reading the introduction.

Part A
Working individually, fill in a list of **benefits of effective teamwork** on one card, and **barriers to effective teamwork** on another card. After five to ten minutes discuss what you have written with one other person, preferably of a different discipline, modifying the entries on the cards as appropriate. (If there is an odd number of participants, there could be one group of three.)

The leader should then ask the whole group to contribute ideas on benefits and barriers to teamwork. This may best be accomplished by asking each person in turn to give their most important item in each category, and for the leader to write them up on the flip-chart in two columns.

It may help to consider the following questions when discussing the ideas:

● Do all team members agree on the benefits and barriers, or are there different responses by individuals or professional groups?

- Do the benefits outweigh the snags for our team?
- Are there particular barriers that we need to address?
- Can the team carry on with the project, or is outside help needed?

If the help of an outside facilitator or consultant is needed, contact should be made with the local Health Authority, or one of the organizations or individuals listed in the 'Useful addresses' section at the end of the book.

Part B

Setting ground rules

As a whole group discuss what ground rules should be established for the practical sessions? Team members may like to consider how seriously they are to take the development of teamwork as demonstrated by such issues as:

- handling interruptions such as phone calls;
- punctuality and regularity of attendance at work and meetings;
- details of confidentiality, what is acceptable and what is unacceptable?
- how do we want to receive feedback about how we work in the team?
- how to ensure that everyone is able to express their point of view?
- what else would help each member to contribute?

Before the end of the meeting, the leader should ask members what they thought about its value.

Facilitator summary

Materials: *Workbook, supply of index cards, flip-chart, pens and paper.*

Activity: **A.** *Revision of recommended reading (5 min).*
Ask participants to work individually and fill in a list on one card of:

(i) Benefits of effective teamwork

(ii) Barriers to effective teamwork (5 min)

Ask individuals to choose someone (preferably from another discipline) to share what they have written.

Ask them to find the most important one in each category (10 min).

Ask them to address the following:

(i) Are there differences between professional groups?

(ii) Do benefits outweigh barriers?

(iii) Are there particular barriers to deal with?

Reconvene the whole group. Ask for a list of benefits of effective teamwork and barriers to effective teamwork. Show these in two columns on flip-chart paper (15 min).

B. *Ask the team to discuss the ground rules they would like to establish for the practical sessions and chart up a list.*
Ensure that each team member is happy with the list, which should be available at each subsequent meeting—either stuck on the wall or a copy distributed to each team member.

Make it clear that changes to the ground rules can be agreed at any time (25 min).

For the next meeting

1. Read Section 1 of the workbook.
2. Write down on the pro forma below, the composition of typical examples of intrinsic and functional teams of which you are a member.
3. List the teams outside the practice or specialist unit of which you are a member.
4. Please bring the completed pro forma to the meeting—it need not be signed.

QUESTIONNAIRE

1. Intrinsic teams

In my contacts with an individual patient, I might need to cooperate with the following members of the team (list by job, not name):

....

....

....

....

....

2. Functional teams

For planning and reviewing patient care or preventive services, or exchanging information, I might need to co-operate with the following members of the team (list by job, not name):

....

....

....

....

....

3. Teamwork external to the practice

As part of my professional work, I am a member of the following teams outside the practice:

....

....

....

....

....

A Questions about teams, goals, and tasks

Section 1: The nature and purpose of teamwork

What are teams?

A team is defined as: **a group of people who make different contributions towards the achievement of a common goal.**

Gilmore *et al.* (1974) described the essential characteristics of teamwork as follows:

1. The members of a team share a common purpose which binds them together and guides their actions.
2. Each member of the team has a clear understanding of his or her own functions, and recognizes common interests.
3. The team works by pooling knowledge, skills, and resources and all members share responsibility for outcome.
4. The effectiveness of a team is related to its capability to carry out its work and to manage itself as an independent group of people.

Team members must constantly ask themselves 'Why am I here?' 'Are we all seeking the same goals?' If not, 'are our aims compatible?' Each team member must be clear about their own job and the contribution it can make to the team goal, and also be aware of the roles of the other team members. People working in a team often assume that they know each other's roles, but do they really? If the team takes on a task, then the whole team must take responsibility if things go wrong—and take credit for success.

13

This is contrary to normal professional work, with its emphasis on personal accountability, but this shared responsibility helps to support team members when things do not turn out well.

The fourth essential characteristic is a great stumbling block to successful team-working. If members of a team have little or no autonomy, they cannot contribute towards decisions, so they have to stall while they refer to higher authority. This can paralyse teamwork. Managers, particularly of nurses and social workers, need to trust their field workers to make the right decisions, within their professional competence, and with due regard to local policies and availability of resources. Managers can help teams to function well by being content with supervision, support and monitoring, not day-to-day control. Team members, particularly doctors, must try to understand these constraints, to which they are less subject, and help the managers and team colleagues to walk this particular tightrope.

This difficulty of divided loyalties is common to all 'matrix organizations' involving several professions and lines of authority. The primary health care team (PHCT) is an example of a matrix organization of unusual complexity, so that the achievement of effective teamwork is a particular challenge, but success is essential for patient care of high quality. The PHCT as an example of a matrix organization is shown in Fig. 3.

In addition to the team members based at the health centre or surgery, other people have such a key role to play that it may be helpful to regard them as team members. This includes the patient and the supporter, and the local community networks, as well as professional and lay helping agencies, who all have a stake in teamwork. Such a group of people are not confined to any one organizational structure, so a system that will accommodate team-working with managed services like nursing or social work, as well as lay people and agencies, has to be designed and run with care. An essential step is to look first at the tasks that need to be done in primary health care and design an organization that will carry out each task, rather than follow the more usual blueprint passed down from above. Fundholding general practices have

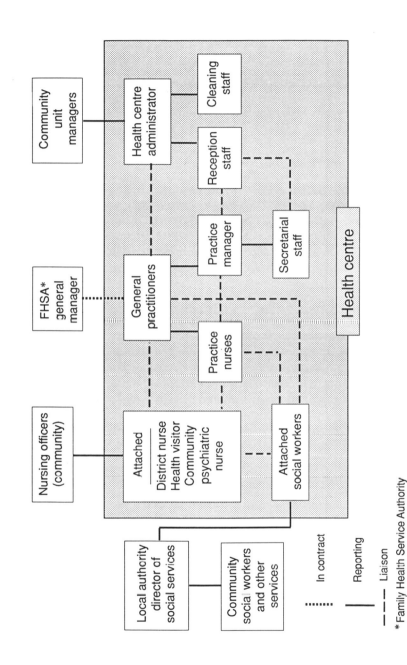

Fig. 3. The team in a health centre is a matrix organization.

Community unit managers

FHSA* general manager

Nursing officers (community)

Health centre administrator

Cleaning staff

Reception staff

Practice manager

Secretarial staff

General practitioners

Health centre

Practice nurses

Attached
District nurse
Health visitor
Community psychiatric nurse

Attached social workers

Local authority director of social services

Community social workers and other services

In contract

Reporting

Liaison

*Family Health Service Authority

greater freedom to design their own organization, but there is a risk of upsetting existing professional balances. Specialist teams in hospital are equally complex, and work in a very large organization, which by its size and complexity alone, makes effective patient care all the more difficult.

Why work in teams?

Much of a doctor's or nurse's time is spent alone with the patient, and this is a feature which patients value highly. But, as mentioned above, many of the important tasks such as maternity care, the care of patients with diabetes or needing home nursing, are obvious candidates for teamwork and shared care. In addition, the role of health care is gradually changing from the former disease-orientation to a wider appreciation of the determinants of ill-health in the lifestyle and the complex physical and psychosocial environment of today. This highlights the need for cooperation across organizational boundaries.

Few objective evaluations have been undertaken of the effectiveness of teamwork over individual care, nor are the boundaries of teamwork clear. Intuitively, people working in teams justify teamwork with reasons such as those listed below:

1. Care given by a group is greater than the sum of individual care.
2. Rare skills are used more appropriately.
3. Team-working encourages continuity of care.
4. The patient gets more efficient and understanding treatment when ill.
5. Peer influence and informal learning within the group raise the standards of care.
6. Team members have more job satisfaction and cope better with failure.
7. Team-working coordinates preventive with curative work.

These statements are difficult to prove unless we can have measurable goals and find out if we achieve them. We hope that participants, at the end of this programme of team-building, will be able to feel more confident that many of these statements are true.

What kinds of team?

The intrinsic team

The central figure, both as the object of care and as an active participant, must be the patient. The lay person or relative providing the main support to the patient in the community comes a close second. Let us take the example from primary healthy care of an elderly woman (living with her daughter) who wakes up with the symptoms of a stroke. The daughter telephones the practice receptionist, who then becomes the key member of the team until the GP takes the message and visits the patient. The GP assesses the problem and decides (jointly with the patient and daughter) that home care would probably be best, and then requests the district nurse to visit and assess the nursing needs. The 'intrinsic' team (Pritchard 1981) now consists of patient, daughter, GP, and district nurse, as shown in Fig. 4. This is the basic building block and action point of flexible teamwork that is re-

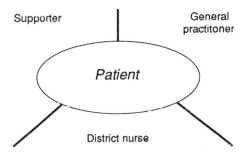

Fig. 4. An example of the intrinsic team.

sponsive to the task in hand, and gets round the difficulty of rigid definitions of who is, and who is not, a team member.

As the tasks change, other people—professional and lay—might be involved, such as a health visitor, a social worker or a lay night attendant. The basic structure of the team would remain centred on the patient and the support network, each with their own special contributions and needs. If the patient is admitted to hospital, a different group of helpers would take over, but the principle of the intrinsic team applies just the same.

Other examples of the intrinsic team in PHC would be focused on the care of women in pregnancy, patients seeing the practice nurse and GP, and patients attending specialist clinics for diabetes, etc., in which more than one professional is involved. This way of looking at teams does not dictate the route by which people obtain care. For example, a patient may first contact the health visitor or district nurse, who is free to consult other team members as appropriate. This way of working is based on the idea of an open and accessible team rather than the alternative of rigid 'delegation' in which the assumption is that all people see the doctor first and are then referred as thought fit.

The functional team

The general practitioner or specialist might have only a vague recollection of which patients were receiving team care at any moment, whereas other professionals would be likely to have a register of their caseloads. In order to share information and awareness of what is going on, all the professionals can benefit by meeting and discussing their shared cases. These meetings need only concern a particular function of teamwork such as home nursing, maternity care, prevention, and screening, etc., and have been called 'functional teams' (Pritchard 1981).

The value of these functional team meetings, which might (in general practice) only occur every six or eight weeks, lies in their review of those patients receiving shared care, and in discussion of policies and procedures. This is an effective form of audit, and the functional team could be seen as a quality circle. Meetings would often involve a review of the case notes held by each professional team member, and this might provide an incentive for access to each other's notes, or in the future, developing an integrated system of records for the team. Clear guidelines would be needed about who enters what in the record, and what access is given to different team members.

If there is no formal structure for these meetings, then only urgent problems will be discussed during chance encounters, and the opportunity for mutual learning and review will be missed. Such meetings can be brief and to the point and only need concern staff directly involved, so little time is wasted and much may be saved.

Functional teams can cover any element of team care that concerns more than one, for example home nursing, social work and maternity care. Practice nursing is another important team function that would benefit from regular review—perhaps with other nurses and the practice manager. The partners and the practice manager would need to meet regularly to discuss and decide upon management issues. The practice manager would have regular meetings with the reception and secretarial staff, preferably attended by a partner with specific responsibilities.

In a hospital setting, say the care of diabetes, the physician might want to meet the dietitian or the ophthalmologist, and not need to involve everybody.

In some practices and departments, different professionals may assume responsibility for an area of management. For example, one doctor might be the 'executive' and liaise with and support the manager. Another professional might be concerned with preventive medicine or aftercare, and attend functional team meetings with the appropriate staff. One doctor might be responsible for finance or budgets, and liaise with the manager and the accountant or finance department. All the partners with a special responsibility would report back to the full team, if appropriate.

The advantages of combining functional teams with specialist leaders would include more efficient involvement of staff in decisions about the work of the unit and considerable saving in time spent at meetings. This is particularly important in larger and specialist units, but smaller units might take some short cuts, for example by having functional team meetings with more than two professions present—for example, doctor, nurse, physiotherapist, and occupational therapist.

The full team

When decisions cannot be taken one-to-one in intrinsic teams or in functional teams, the full team needs to meet. Major issues of policy such as a move to a new building, introducing new services, or discussing the annual report and future plans are examples: Or issues such as holiday rotas and an annual party might need the full team. If this policy is followed, much time and boredom will be saved. Teamwork often gets a bad name from long meetings about topics which only concern a few, so people chat in small groups or leave early and chaos reigns. If meetings of the full team are regular, but infrequent, and have a salient agenda, then people will find them worthwhile. Meetings are considered further in Section 5 (pp. 56–67).

Size of teams

A PHC team of five full-time partners might have ten employed staff and six to ten attached staff. This results in a full team size of 25. If some are part-time, the number might be 35, so that in a one-hour meeting each would be lucky to have two minutes to speak. This is a long way from the ideal of dialogue, in which two people share the talking and listening time equally. Experience has shown that teams of more than 20 have serious problems of communication. Belbin (1981) regards teams of ten as too large for effective decision making, and settles for a team of six members as ideal.

Some practices have found that the 'firm' system works well—for example a practice of six GPs could work as two firms of three, each with their own employed and attached staff, coordinated by the practice manager. Some go even further with each GP having an individual secretary or receptionist, and a nominated practice nurse and attached staff (who might work with more than one GP). These structural arrangements combine the 'small is beautiful' and personal care notions, with the advantages of a larger unit. Likewise, the intrinsic and functional team concept works with teams of around three to six people. Each practice needs to decide on its own structure, whether personal lists are used and the way intrinsic and functional teams are organized. This is part of the practical exercise that follows.

Why develop team working?

In the early days of setting up teams in the British National Health Service (NHS), the assumption was that teamwork would occur in primary health care if the district nurses and health visitors were attached to general practices. Indeed, it sometimes did, but as the Harding–Frost (DHSS 1981) report revealed, teamwork from the viewpoint of nurses was very unsatisfactory. The report recommended that teamwork should be developed by educational means. Some notable initiatives have occurred, and many excellent examples of teamwork are known. But if we are to achieve a general level of quality of teamwork that would satisfy patients, doctors and other staff as well as health authorities (and trusts), and the flexibility to cope with change, then there must be scope for learning.

The changing and increasing demands made upon health care services to meet today's needs have been mentioned. This implies that people's roles must change too. New skills are needed both to treat patients and to coordinate the care of patients. So teamwork must be open to change. The old ways may, or may not, be appropriate. Every team needs to be a 'learning organization' (Senge 1992; Swieringa and Wierdsma 1992) (see Section 14, p. 123).

Fortunately, the basic theory and practice of teamwork has been firmly established and validated, both in industry and in public services such as primary and secondary health care. There is no need to reinvent the wheel. The example chosen as the basis of this workbook was developed at the Sloan School of Management of the Massachusetts Institute of Technology (MIT) in the 1970s (Rubin and Beckhard 1972; Rubin *et al.* 1975; Plovnick *et al.* 1978), and has been thoroughly tested in health care settings in the USA and in the UK.

Learning exercise 1: What are teams, and why work in them? Kinds of team

Aim: To explore the nature and purpose of teamwork.

Objectives: By the end of the session participants will have:

(1) read the relevant section of recommended reading;
(2) made clear to themselves, and to each other, the kinds of teams of which they are part;
(3) explored their most successful ways of working in teams;
(4) **Optional**—produced a 'map' of all sub-teams and outside teams.

If necessary allow ten minutes for reading Section 1 and completing the pro forma.

Working in groups of two or three (of different disciplines), start by sharing the information in the pro forma, and discussing the kinds of team that you are part of, and how these teams function, and relate to each other.

After about 30 minutes come back to the full group to discuss ideas about the structure and function of teams that have arisen in your small groups. As with the previous exercise the facilitator could ask for contributions in turn. What are the most successful ways of working in teams for your practice?

As a sub-project a team member could collect the pro formas (unsigned) and collate them in order to produce a 'map' of all the sub-teams within the unit, and outside teams. This could be shown to all team members, and discussed later.

Facilitator summary

Materials: *Flip-chart, paper*

Activity: *Revision of recommended reading (10 min)*

Ask participants to divide into sets of two or three people of different disciplines.

Ask that they share results shown on the pro forma (10 min).

Specifically ask them to discuss the kinds of team of which they are part and how these teams function and relate to each other (20 min).

Re-form the full group. Ask for what was discussed in small groups. Summarize this on flip-chart paper emphasizing the most successful ways of working in teams (20 min).

Optional task requires extra time—collect unsigned pro formas and suggest that a team member (or members) collates the information to map all sub-teams and outside teams. This can then be shared with all members.

For the next meeting

Please read Section 2 of the workbook (pp. 32–6), and complete a 'team diagnostic instrument', as shown in subsequent pages. Preferably these pages should be photocopied, so that they could be collected (unsigned) and collated in confidence, in order to present the overall 'team diagnosis' at the next meeting.

This is an important exercise, and one that some people may be reluctant to complete. This would reflect how 'safe' team members felt in describing their perceptions of the team. Both the importance of filling in the questionnaire and also its confidential nature should be stressed.

CONFIDENTIAL QUESTIONNAIRE ON TEAM WORKING—PART 1

1. Team goals

Please read both statements, and ring one letter which seems closest to the way your team functions:

Statement I 'I often wonder why we work as a team. We seem to spend a lot of time and energy doing things which I do not think important, rather than concentrating on things which help us to achieve our main goals'.

> a. Just like statement I
> b. More like I than II
> c. In between I and II
> d. More like II than I
> e. Just like statement II

Statement II 'I am very clear about what our team is trying to achieve, and we all put our efforts into it. Whenever a question arises about what needs doing we are able to get our priorities right by referring back to our main goals.'

Describe below any examples of situations in your team which illustrate your response to this question:

....

....

....

2. My job (role)

Please read both statements, and ring one letter which seems closest to the way your team functions:

Statement I 'Situations often arise in my job where I am uncertain what I am supposed to do. I am often not sure when something is my responsibility or someone else's. We never discuss what each of us thinks he or she, and other members of the team could or should do for best results.'

        a. Just like statement I
        b. More like I than II
        c. In between I and II
        d. More like II than I
        e. Just like statement II

Statement II 'In almost every situation I am sure about what are my responsibilities, and what other team members are supposed to be doing. When a query arises, we discuss where we each think our responsibilities lie.'

Examples:

....

....

....

3. How things get done here–procedures

Participation

Please read both statements, and ring one letter which seems closest to the way your team functions:

Statement I 'When some people try to join in a discussion, they are often interrupted, or their suggestions are ignored. People seem to pay attention to some team members, but not to others. Some people seem to do most of the talking, while others don't participate much or at all.'

      a. Just like statement I
      b. More like I than II
      c. In between I and II
      d. More like II than I
      e. Just like statement II

Statement II 'Everyone gets a chance to speak and to influence the discussion. We listen to everyone's contribution. No one is ignored. Everyone is drawn into the discussion.'

Examples:

....

....

....

Decisions

Please read both statements, and ring one letter which seems closest to the way your team functions:

Statement I 'After a discussion I often wonder what took place, and what is supposed to happen next. If I am expected to do something, I often do not agree with the task assigned to me. It seems that problems keep coming up for discussion when I thought we had decided about them.'

      a. Just like statement I
      b. More like I than II
      c. In between I and II
      d. More like II than I
      e. Just like statement II

Statement II 'When we discuss a problem, I usually understand exactly what the issue is, and what we have decided to do about it, and what are my responsibilities. Decisions made by the team are effectively carried out by team members.'

Examples:

....

....

....

Managing conflict

Please note that this is a different style of question.

First read all the statements, and ring the one which most closely describes the situation in your team.

When a disagreement arises in the team:

a. We assume it is best not to let it get personal, so we let it pass and hope it will soon be forgotten. If feelings start to get heated, we try to cool things down by making the least of the disagreement (for example 'there is no point in getting angry, so let's forget it').

b. We often end the disagreement when someone takes charge and makes a decision, and it is not discussed further.

c. We try to come to an agreement somewhere between the two conflicting positions. In other words we compromise, so everyone gains a little and loses a little and so we end the disagreement.

d. We try to get the disagreeing parties together and let them talk through their points of view, until each can see some sense in the other's ideas. Then we try to reach an agreement which makes sense to everyone.

Examples:

....

....

....

4. What it feels like to work in this team

Availability

Please read both statements, and ring one letter which seems closest to the way your team functions:

Statement I 'When you need to get hold of another team member, it is really difficult. Either they are not here, or they haven't got time to talk to you. But they seem to find time for other things.'

        a. Just like statement I
        b. More like I than II
        c. In between I and II
        d. More like II than I
        e. Just like statement II

Statement II 'When you have a question, or need some help from another team member, there is no problem in getting hold of anyone. People go out of their way to be available to each other. I have no difficulty talking to anyone on the team.'

Examples:

....

....

....

Mutual support

Please read both statements, and ring one letter which seems closest to the way your team functions:

Statement I 'This job is really frustrating. People do not seem to be concerned with helping others to get the job done. They go their own way. But if you try to do something different, or make a mistake, you get no help or support.'

Ring one letter which seems closest to the way your team functions:

  a. Just like statement I
  b. More like I than II
  c. In between I and II
  d. More like II than I
  e. Just like statement II

Statement II 'I really like my job, and working in this team. The team encourages you to take responsibility. Other team members appreciate your efforts, and help when things are not going well. We really pull together in this team.'

Examples:

....

....

Further comments:

....

....

Thank you for completing this questionnaire. Please hand it in, unsigned, to the nominated collator in good time before the next meeting.

Acknowledgement: This questionnaire is a modified version of a *Health team diagnostic instrument* published in Plovnick, M., Fry, R., and Rubin, I. (1978) *Managing health care delivery. A training program for primary care physicians.* Ballinger Publishing Co., Cambridge, Mass.

Section 2: Team diagnosis

How are we doing as a team?

Having looked at the sort of team structure that suits our own situation and the people involved, the next step is a bolder one. We must ask ourselves:

1. **How good is our team? Can we measure its quality?**
2. **Can we identify our strong points as well as our weaknesses?**

We can start to answer these questions by applying a 'diagnostic instrument'—like a stethoscope—to our team. Is its heart beating strongly? Are there some pathological signs or murmurs? Experience from the United States (Rubin *et al.* 1975) showed that there were four main factors involved in the coordination of primary care, and these are listed below.

Goals: Do all team members share the same goals?

General practitioners and specialists may see their work in quite a different light compared to—say—nurses or lay staff. Some doctors focus mainly on the treatment of medical diseases—the 'doctor-centred' doctor described by Byrne and Long (1976). This is no bad thing, as the main functions of a GP are to detect, treat, and, if necessary, refer patients with serious or life-threatening illnesses. At the other end of the spectrum is the 'patient-centred' doctor, who is more concerned with the patient's personal and psychosocial problems. If these differences of approach exist within one profession, much wider discrepancies are likely to exist between—say—doctors and nurses or social workers.

People working in health care teams are busy and practical. They are primarily concerned with getting the job done. So, once our goals are clear, we can get on with the task. Following the question 'why are we here?' comes 'what is the task for this particular patient?' Until this is decided, we are in no position to consider who should do it, nor how it should be done. Consequently, the key message of team-building is to ask the right questions in the right order. For example:

1. What are our goals? What is the task? Does it need teamwork?

2. What are our various roles in the team? Who will carry out the task?

3. What are the agreed procedures for successful teamwork? How do we carry out and evaluate the team tasks?

4. Are our interpersonal relationships as good as possible? Is team effectiveness threatened by unresolved conflict?

For team-building to be effective, experience in many settings has shown the advantages of this order of approach. By focusing on goals, tasks, roles and procedures, we build a solid basis for cooperative teamwork and mutual trust, so that harmonious interpersonal relationships are likely to develop. The first three categories are where we have to look for factors that lead to effective teamwork. Poor interpersonal relationships may often be a symptom of failure to get the first three factors right. After all, what better way is there of building respect than working together successfully? If, however, we start with discussing how we could get on better together, or focus on personalities and conflicts, then we may never get round to discussing goals and tasks, bearing in mind the very short time that can be set aside for communicating. If conflict becomes an issue, team members could read section 8 and consider whether they needed help from an outside facilitator.

Learning exercise 2: Applying a questionnaire

Applying a questionnaire as a diagnostic instrument to our own team is done to find out where we are strong, and where there are opportunities for improvement.

Aim:
To explore the operation of the defined PHC team.

Objectives:
By the end of the session participants will have:

(1) read the relevant section of recommended reading;

(2) discussed the results from the completed confidential questionnaire;

(3) decided which of the following should take greatest priority:
    (a) goals and tasks
    (b) roles
    (c) procedures
    (d) interpersonal relationships

(4) decided which of these needs greatest time and effort.

Feedback of results from the team 'diagnostic instrument'

The collator will have summarized all the questionnaire responses on to a single sheet, and also listed (or summarized) the comments under each heading. The summary and comments will be given to all the participants, if possible in advance of the meeting. Only the collator will see the questionnaires, which are confidential. The participants will be free to discuss the responses openly. They are classified under the four headings listed in Section 2, that is to say goals/tasks, roles, procedures, and interpersonal relationships. Each of these topics will be taken in turn in later sessions, so only the diagnosis need be discussed and the priorities for future attention, not the 'treatment' itself.

Overleaf is a blank summary sheet (Fig. 5) for the collator to block in the relevant square boldly, so that the results can be seen at a glance. If the bulk of the responses are to the right of the figures, that represents satisfactory team working (and vice versa).

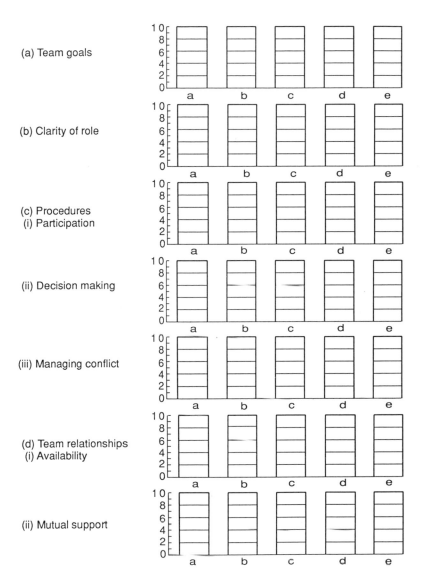

(a) Team goals

(b) Clarity of role

(c) Procedures
    (i) Participation

(ii) Decision making

(iii) Managing conflict

(d) Team relationships
    (i) Availability

(ii) Mutual support

Fig. 5. A blank team diagnostic summary sheet.

Particular attention should be given to the areas of teamwork that stand out as satisfactory and unsatisfactory, so that the team can see what is going well, before facing up to the areas of teamwork that fall short.

This session must concentrate on diagnosis, not treatment. That can come later in the appropriate section. The easy option is to jump to treatment before making a diagnosis, collecting and assessing information, and then looking at options for treatment.

An example of a completed team summary is shown in Fig. 6 (page 37).

Comment on example of team diagnosis

Figure 6 shows all but one team member giving positive responses, and half the team members (on average) giving optimum responses—an unusually high level. However, one team member (not necessarily the same one) was neutral or negative. The best area seemed to be mutual support, and the least good being the management of conflict. One individual stood out as feeling isolated from participation in the team, and critical of procedures for decision making and managing conflict. But what were their standards and expectations, and how could the more isolated members be brought on board? A repeat of the diagnosis at the end of the development process might reveal interesting changes.

Some possible questions for discussion.

- Do we accept the logical order of the questions and the sessions?
- Should we focus first on goals and tasks, or start with—say—procedures or interpersonal relationships?
- What does the questionnaire reveal that we do well? Do we all agree?
- How could we do better? Should we spend more time on the areas where there is scope for improvement?

At the close of the meeting, the leader should ask for views as to its usefulness, and the value of the 'diagnostic instrument'.

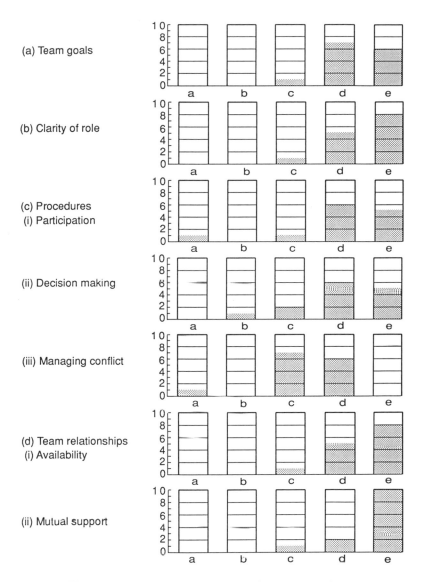

(a) Team goals

(b) Clarity of role

(c) Procedures
(i) Participation

(ii) Decision making

(iii) Managing conflict

(d) Team relationships
(i) Availability

(ii) Mutual support

Fig. 6. A completed team diagnostic summary sheet.

Facilitator summary

Materials: *It is important for the session that the confidential questionnaires have been collated including a list of comments under each heading. A copy can then be circulated to participants. Questionnaires will only be seen by the collator.*

Activity: *Emphasize that the exercise is diagnostic, that is it is measuring areas of teamwork to discover which are satisfactory and which are unsatisfactory. It is not about tackling any identified problems.*
Ask the following questions, possibly by 'headlining' them on flip-chart paper:

(i)   What does the questionnaire reveal that we do well?

(ii) Should we focus first on goals and tasks, roles, procedures, or interpersonal relationships.

(iii) Should we spend more time on the areas where-there is scope for improvement?

For the next meeting

Please read Section 3 of the workbook, and write down on one or more cards the answers to the questions shown below (not more than three answers on each card):

1. What are my own personal goals at work—in the medium term (say one to two years)?

2. What do I see as goals for the team in the medium term (say one to two years); and the dates for their achievement?

3. What is my own 'ideal vision' of how I would like the department or practice to be in five years from now? Present constraints should be disregarded but allowance made for how I think the future will look in five years.

These cards should be brought to the next meeting for discussion in small groups. They will not be collected nor seen by anyone else.

Section 3: Team goals and tasks

What are we trying to achieve?

Goal setting should be seen as a means to an end rather than an end in itself, and so it is worth considering a few questions before setting out to define some goals of our own.

Why set goals?

What will they do for me and the team? The answer will depend on the particular goal and particular team, but some of the reasons given by teams are as follows.

1. Goals define a direction to go in and so make it easier to decide what is best to do next.
2. For the team, goals will make that direction explicit and so create a common understanding.
3. Goals can help to define who is responsible for what.
4. Goals can be a help to motivate us to do our jobs more-effectively, since we are all clear about what we are trying to achieve.

How to set goals?

Two alternative approaches, which may lead to totally different kinds of goal, can be distinguished as follows:

1. We can look at what we are doing now and think about how that might change over a period of time. This is goal setting by **extrapolation**.

2. We can imagine, in detail, how things might work in an ideal world, ignoring the constraints that we normally take for granted. This is goal setting by **envisioning**.

The first method will lead us to evolutionary improvement: the second may result in a more radical change of course. Eventually we must come back from our ideal world to the reality of today. Our vision may seem unrealistic, but barriers that now seem unsurmountable may disappear, or we may find a completely different route to our goal. Whether we set goals by extrapolation or envisioning, we need to be aware of which method we are using and of the consequences of using that method.

Criteria for effective goals

All goals are not equally effective in achieving what we want, so how do we frame goals that work best? Some important characteristics of effective goals are as follows:

Goals should be positively framed. It is very difficult to work to negative objectives. For instance, a negative goal might be 'to stop wasting my time by poorly conducted meetings and unpunctuality'. A positive goal might be 'to ensure the efficient use of team time by conducting meetings briskly and punctually'.

Goals should be challenging but realistic. In order to motivate not demoralize, goals should be set at an appropriate level.

Goals should be within our capability. A personal or team goal is less likely to be effective if it is highly dependant on outside resources. It may be possible to reframe the goal to cover the part we control.

Goals should be specific and measurable. We must be able to tell when we have achieved our goal.

Goals should be agreed.   All those who are concerned with the results, and who have to do the work to achieve them, should agree on the goals.

Goals should be acceptable.   Goals must be acceptable to us in the context of our personal and professional values, and our other activities, both within and outside our working lives.

Types of goal

Goals may be 'high-level' ones, involving the purposes of medical care, or the quality of life of sick people, or the meaning of illness. Or they may be everyday ones, like the purpose of a meeting. Unless people can agree why they are devoting their time to a meeting, conflict and frustration are inevitable. One advantage of the team structure proposed earlier is that meetings of intrinsic and functional teams have a much clearer purpose than the larger team meetings.

Another way of distinguishing types of goal is to identify **end goals** and the **process goals** needed to achieve them.

An **end goal** is defined in terms of an external target, whether that be a measure of patient (or staff) satisfaction, or reaching a screening target, or persuading 20 per cent of our smoking patients to give up, or being (measurably) the best practice in the district. This type of goal is partly outside the control of the team and so we may fail to meet it however good we are.

A **process goal** is defined within the team and relates to the way we work, and is entirely within our control. For example, we could work through this book to the end; or we could set up a 'Give up Smoking' clinic, in order to work towards the end goal mentioned above.

It is worth setting both types of goal on the basis that if we continue to meet our process goals (and we are not too unlucky) we will also realize our end goals. If, however, we focus only on an end goal, failure will be more catastrophic, as we have no fall-back position. Failure to meet a goal is hurtful, whereas success breeds success.

How to define explicit goals

If you ask people about their goals, they may be at a loss for words. We tend to be reticent about our strong beliefs and the moral and ethical values that inspire them, as if the light of day will harm them. But nothing is so helpful to a team in developing its identity and morale as the discovery of shared goals. Identifying when goals are not shared, or are in direct conflict, is equally important, just as the driver needs to learn about crossroads and red traffic lights. But we need to concentrate on positive goals, on which we agree, so that we can make progress.

Do all team members have compatible goals?

Unless goals are spelled out, we do not appreciate how much they differ. We then stumble over the obstacles that incompatibility can cause. Some partners may aim at maximizing their income, some at being needed by their patients. Doctors may be totally immersed in their job, to the exclusion of nearly everything else. But they cannot expect a part-time receptionist to have the same attitude. Doctors and nurses train and socialize in the same in-stitutions, and share some of the same work culture. Social workers, however, usually train and work in a different culture and kind of organization. Goal conflicts are much more likely to arise as a consequence. Yet 'broad spectrum' cooperation is of critical importance in health care today. It is achievable, but it requires effort and understanding. (See Clare and Corney 1982; Huntington 1981a; Ratoff *et al.* 1974.)

Setting priorities for tasks in terms of urgency and importance

Once we have made our goals and tasks explicit, the next stage is to decide the order of action. This will be considered further in Section 5.

Learning exercise 3: Setting positive individual goals, comparing them with team goals, and negotiating a way forward

Aim: To set positive individual goals, compare them with team goals and negotiate a way forward.

Objectives: By the end of the session participants will have:

(1) read the relevant section of recommended reading;

(2) compared individual goals with other group members;

(3) discussed team goals and listed what they have in common with individual goals;

(4) discussed individual visions of the future;

(5) **Optional**—produced a 'map' of an ideal future that is a product of consensus.

If necessary allow 10 minutes to read Section 3 of the workbook and complete the questions at the end of Section 2.

Working in groups of two or three (of different disciplines), discuss and compare your individual goals and whether they are the same, overlap or are in opposition to those of other members of your group. Then consider the team goals and visions, and discuss what they have in common. Try to keep the discussion to the goals themselves, not how to achieve them. That comes at a later session (20 min).

Re-form the main group and describe some of the goals that were shared and some that were in conflict, in each of the small groups (20 min).

Next, people from each group should describe some of their visions for the future. A nominated member should write these down, and later, as a sub-project, try to devise a 'map' of an ideal future that most participants would share, and put this up on the wall. This map is just a vision of the future. How we get there is another question! A note should also be kept of shared and conflicting goals for future discussions (15 min).

Before closing the session, the leader will ask for views of its usefulness.

Facilitator summary

Materials: *Flip-chart paper, previous 'takeaway results'*

Activity: *Revision of recommended reading (10 min)*

Divide into sets of two or three people of different disciplines

(i) Ask participants to discuss and compare individual goals with sub-group members, noting similarities and differences.

(ii) Do the same with team goals and visions trying to find what they have in common (15 min).

Re-form main group. Ask for descriptions of shared goals and conflicting goals. Note these on flip-chart paper (20 min).

Ask for each participant's vision for the future. Write these on flip-chart paper (15 min).

Optional *(requires extra time) Produce a 'map' of an ideal future of the team which all team members can agree.*

For the next meeting

Please read Section 4 of the workbook, and write down on a card, in less than 20 words, what you consider to be the most important part of your professional role. Head the card with your job, but not your name. A member of each professional group will collect their colleagues' cards before the next meeting. Team members should also write down (on a separate card to bring to the meeting, not for collection), what parts of their job they think they do well. Please give the completed card to a member of your discipline for summarizing before the meeting.

Write on card for collection.

My job is ....

The most important part of my professional role is

....

....

....

....

Please complete this card and bring it to the next meeting (not for collection).

These are the parts of my job that I think I do well:

....

....

....

....

B   Who does what in our team

Section 4: Roles within the team

Who does what in our team?

Modern health care requires a multiplicity of skills, some of which are specific to one profession, and some, such as counselling and communicating or health education, may be common to several professions.

All team members are contributing of their best, and this must be reflected in equality of status, not a hierarchy based on pay. The key to effective teamwork is for everyone's work to be **valued**, and this value must be appreciated by all the members of the team. For this to happen, each team member must have a clear perception of their own role and must also be aware of each other's role. Many professional roles are changing, resulting in role-uncertainty and lack of confidence. To be motivated for high performance, people must have an infectious enthusiasm for the work they are doing (Vaill 1982).

Team members might be expected to acquire a clear idea of what the others do, just by working together. But this does not necessarily happen. People are reticent about their own view of their role, and may go on accepting inappropriate expectations or referrals without protest. Asking the GP to describe the health visitor's or social worker's role may produce answers that are hilarious or hurtful, but it is a step towards mutual understanding and esteem.

Can some of the skills that were traditionally part of medicine, such as diagnosis or prescribing, be shared with other professions? The practice nurse takes on many tasks which doctors used to do, such as taking blood pressure, syringing ears and suturing. But does the nurse accept this as 'job enrichment', or is it just the doctor passing on the boring tasks? Similarly, the nurse in hospital carries out many tasks that were the doctor's, as well as undertaking new technical tasks such as intensive care. The implication (as seen in industry) is that the doctor, being paid more, should delegate to the less well-paid and thus save money. This argument may make economic sense, but it is regarding the nurse as of lower status and this does not make for good teamwork. Can doctors bring themselves to discuss this openly, by asking nurses and other staff what jobs they would like to do more or less often, and which tasks they do not regard as part of their professional role?

'Role-specification' (a detailed description of what a professional does, or is expected to do), and the boundaries between roles in health care are far from clear. For example, in PHC, there may be overlap in the roles of the health visitor and social worker; the GP, the district nurse and the practice nurse; the GP and the midwife; and the practice manager and the 'executive' GP. These overlaps can give rise to confusion and ill-will, but often this is hidden so that the conflict takes other forms. Once confidence is established, considerable flexibility of role can be accepted, so that if the role expectations of an individual are not in tune with what other members expect, then some give-and-take or 'role negotiation' is possible. This capacity to perceive and change role boundaries is one of the key issues in team-building. During periods of turbulent change in society and in health service organization, people tend to feel anxious for their professional future and raise interprofessional barriers—just when the need for effective teamwork is all the stronger.

How people work together

When people first meet with a view to working together, the relationship develops through several stages. The first is sharing information about themselves, what they can offer and their expectations of each other. This information may start with a job description, a *curriculum vitae*, and an interview. Or it may start more abruptly, when a new staff member is posted to the team. The more clearly the mutual expectations are expressed, the less uncertainty there will be in the relationship, and some prediction of behaviour will be possible. The next stage is a commitment to shared expectations and a clearer definition of roles. As people work together, they get to know how each will react in a wider range of situations, and if all goes well, the working relationship becomes stable and productive. For example, if a new staff nurse joins the team, there will be an early period of adjustment, when the existing team compares her to her predecessor, and the nurse sees how the new group measures up to her expectations based on past experience. Each will need to show that the new relationship will be different and better. In time the unique features of each individual and each team will be seen in a truer light.

Role negotiation

The third stage is to question whether our roles meet other people's expectations, and if they do not, to negotiate changes in our role. Even in an ideal team, circumstances will arise that disrupt the stability, and put new strains on the relationship. For example, one staff member may leave so that extra work is put on those remaining, or a particularly upsetting case may go wrong, or a team member may go on a course and return with changed expectations that are not shared. This new situation can be recognized for what it is, and a renegotiation of expectations will result in a return to the previous stable and productive phase. Or the relationship may become ambiguous—they can no longer be sure of each other—with resulting anxiety and resentment about working together. This leads to a painful point of decision 'the crunch', with three possible paths to take.

The first path is to return to the way things were before (that is to ignore that there are new circumstances) but this is only patching up the team relationship. The second is for someone to opt out or leave in a huff, which may be needless as well as painful. The third way is to renegotiate the expectations and behaviour, so that a new equilibrium is established to meet the changed circumstances. For example, a health visitor may have a greatly increased case-load and be unable to undertake geriatric screening which she had done willingly before; or key staff in a hospital team may leave and replacement be disallowed, with serious effects on teamwork.

In a flexible team, a crisis can be avoided and other options sought by a process of negotiation. In the first example, the practice nurse might do some of the work, with a period of induction training by the health visitor and other team members, as appropriate. In the second example, a solution may have to be found within the team, however unsatisfactory. Learning these problem-solving and negotiating skills as a group will strengthen the team and give it more confidence to face future uncertainties. The solution to the problem may indeed be for a staff member to leave, but if this conclusion is reached after a period of re-negotiation, then it will be less hurtful.

Practical steps

To summarize, we can ask ourselves five questions:

1. What do we perceive as our own professional role?
2. What do we perceive as other team members' professional roles?
3. Are these perceptions true and realistic? If not, can we correct faulty perceptions?
4. Do our own roles meet what other team members need and expect of us?
5. If this is not so, what can we do to change ourselves, and do others need to change too?

The first four steps are diagnostic, the fifth means learning to behave differently following role negotiation. This is a delicate area, close to people's feelings of personal and professional worth, and needs to be approached with care and sensitivity in a spirit of give-and-take, not blame. The process, like marriage guidance, can be helped by writing messages to each other. These are known as role messages, and they can be about the roles of members of a profession in general, or they can be specific, between two individuals.

General role messages

An example of a general role message is when a doctor says that he or she would like social workers to respond more quickly when a suspected case of child abuse is notified; or for a district nurse to wish that general practitioners would spend more time visiting cases being nursed at home, rather than leave all the decisions to the nurse. This kind of role negotiation is relatively painless, but it is less effective than a direct message to an individual with an ensuing dialogue.

Individual role messages

These work better with a set format, which includes why you want a change and what changes, of which an example follows:

To: Jack Roberts (GP)

From: Fiona Jackson (Practice Nurse or Staff Nurse)

In order to help me make a success of the cardiovascular disease prevention programme, I *need you to do*:

more of: the follow-up of patients who default on treatment;

the same: advising people known to be at risk;

less of: expecting me to be able to influence people who have been obese for a long time.

Note that every category need not be filled in, and if you do not want anything to change, fill in 'the same of everything'.

At its most extreme, every team member might want to send a role message, or even several messages, to every other team member. In a team of eleven, everyone would have to send and receive ten messages or more. This would mean 100 or more messages and subsequent dialogue. (A short cut is suggested in the practical exercises, and the subsequent section can be regarded as a separate exercise to be undertaken when convenient.)

Role negotiation one-to-one

The next stage, after individual role messages have been sent, is for the sender and receiver to meet and for the message to be explained and clarified. The receiver can then respond in a number of ways, for example:

1. That is a good idea. I will do it.
2. I do not have the time to do that, but I will see if someone else (for example a trainee, student, or secretary) will undertake it.
3. I cannot do what you suggest, but I can see another way round your problem that we might discuss.

The two parties would then discuss the issues, negotiate a solution, and come up with a 'contract' (ideally written down) that covers the nature of the problem and what each person would do. This stresses the mutuality of role negotiation. It is not just one person telling another that they must change, but an agreement that both will change in order to deal with the task or problem. This negotiation may be an entirely private matter between two professionals, or it may involve the whole team, in which case the new 'contract' could be discussed at a meeting. This cannot all happen at one session, as it is a continuing process for dealing with changing circumstances. It should be an integral part of team management, and time should be scheduled for it.

For role negotiation to succeed, there must be a climate of mutual trust. Team members need to express the esteem and value of each other's contribution, rather than dwell too much on shortcomings. A good start is to look at what people do well in their job.

Learning exercise 4: Role description and negotiation

Defining our jobs, what we do well, and which parts need negotiation.

Aim: To explore perceptions of professional roles.

Objectives: By the end of the session participants will have:

(1) read the relevant recommended reading and completed the question cards;
(2) described the part(s) of the job that they do well;
(3) described what they think other members of the group do well;
(4) discussed any differences in perceptions between (2) and (3).

If necessary allow 10 minutes for reading Section 4 and filling in the pro forma at the end of Section 3. A representative of each discipline should spend 5 minutes summarizing what colleagues have written down as the most important part of their own role, as they see it.

Working in multidisciplinary groups of two to four, take turns to describe what part of your job you think you do well. Then take turns again to say what you think members of the other disciplines in the group do well. Any agreements and differences between these sets of perceptions should be discussed in the small groups. (25 minutes).

Re-form the full group and give a brief report of what happened in each small group. The leader should first try to focus the discussion, in the light of the messages from the small groups, on the positive aspects of how people see each others' contributions; then on the differences in role perception, and whether any negotiation or modification of roles is needed.

Sub-project on further role negotiation

If time does not allow a full exploration of these issues, or if there is evidence of serious role conflict, an option would be to set up an extra session on role negotiation. If the problem is restricted to a few individuals or disciplines, they could arrange their own session, or meet one-to-one. Before this extra session, participants should be invited to write 'role messages' to each other, as described above.

A role message works best if it is in a very specific form in order to minimize conflict. In the example quoted earlier, a doctor may send a message to a social worker requesting that he or she (or the office) responds more promptly (that is not more than 24 hours) to requests to visit cases of suspected child abuse. The reason would be that the doctor thinks that the child's life is at risk and cannot stand the anxiety of inaction, adding that when the request is made personally to a named social worker, there is usually less of a problem. This is an example of the social worker's behaviour being controlled from the office (outside the team domain), and possibly of excessive caseload. A discussion might result in the adoption of a procedure for cases considered to be urgent, or alternative options sought in order to get action, such as informing the police or a voluntary agency.

If the constraint is a bureaucratic one, the team might show solidarity and support the professional in their conflict, or find some other way around the log jam. The method helps to avoid the conflict becoming personal by exploring the reasons for it objectively and positively, and offering something in return. The social worker's response might be that the doctor is more concerned with the child, rather than the family as a whole, and some 'give and take' might resolve the issue.

Members can also be invited to discuss, from their own experience, examples of role conflicts (not personal conflicts) that have occurred, and how they were dealt with. They can try to confine any discussion to role conflicts, as conflict in the broader context is discussed later.

Facilitator summary

Materials: *Nil*

Activity: *Revision of recommended reading and completion of 'job role' cards (10 min).*

Ask participants to split into single discipline sets. Each discipline to summarize what colleagues have written as their most important role (5 min).

Ask participants to form into multidisciplinary sets of two to four.
Ask each set member in turn to state:

  (i)   *What part of their job they think they do well;*
  (ii) *what they think members of the other disciplines in the group do well;*

  (iii) *Highlight and discuss any difficulties (25 min);*
        Re-form large group. Ask for a summary of what happened in each group. Focus discussion on:

  (i)   *Positive aspects of participants' perceptions;*

  (ii) *Differences in role perception;*

  (iii) *Whether any negotiation or modification is needed (20 min).*

Optional *(needs extra time). An extra (subsequent) session may be needed to continue negotiation of roles.*

For the next session

Please read Section 5 of the workbook (pp. 56–65), and write down on a card what you regard as the most important issue or issues facing the team (not more than three and each issue on a separate card), and hand them, unsigned, to a nominated person for collation.

C How we get things done here

Section 5: Meetings, decisions, procedures, and use of time

Who takes decisions and how?

Health care teams have much in common with industrial team settings, and each can learn from the other. However, there are also differences to bear in mind. For example, the interplay of professional roles is very complex indeed. Attached staff have managers outside the team, who may have very different goals. Doctors may feel the burden of legal responsibility for their decisions, even if some are team decisions. They feel that the buck stops with them, and that time presses particularly hard on them. These perceptions may affect the way they make decisions, and make them feel isolated, rather than draw support from other team members. As a result they may appear to be autocratic, and to assume a monopoly of decision making. This is hard on other professional staff like nurses, social workers, and the unit secretary or manager, all of whom should have autonomy in their own field, and should have the opportunity to influence team decisions.

Doctors, in common with other health professionals, do indeed carry a heavy load of responsibility, but one of the essential characteristics of teamwork is a shared responsibility for outcome. This helps to lessen the professional isolation and to make perceived failure easier to bear. All team members may feel they are on a slippery slope, because all patients have to die one day, and they may interpret death as failure. Doctors and nurses all like to see their patients' good health, freedom from pain and survival as key goals that motivate their every action. This is, of course, Utopian but what alternatives do they have? They find it difficult to modify these laudable goals for fear of becoming callous and uncaring about death. Even when they have to accept the inevitability of pain and death, they are still surrounded by much grief and sorrow. These characteristics of health professionals make a sharing of goals and decisions all the more imperative. Similarly, a sharing of tasks can lessen the distress they cause, for example in primary health care, evening visits to the terminally ill and follow-up bereavement visits might be shared between two members of the team. Issues like death and bereavement may be difficult to discuss between team members, until a climate of mutual trust has developed, and the setting is regarded as 'safe'.

The doctor as manager of the practice or department

Doctors tend to be decisive when faced with an individual patient's problem, and to be good managers of clinical problems, but perhaps when managing an organization, like the practice or department, the problems and techniques are different. Many doctors want to avoid conflict with their peers, and so avoid managing actively with an eye to the future. They can do this by avoiding making decisions, or by failing to carry out the decisions that have been made. This desire to avoid conflict is understandable, but may drive it underground, and result in less effective teamwork.

Doctors often have a responsibility to engage and manage some of the team staff, and in general practice, the premises. The relationship within the team is entirely different—namely one of cooperation and mutual regard. This means that doctors will have to realize that other team members are managing their patch as well. Some may indeed have training in management. They all share the responsibility for the way the team as a whole is seen by patients, by professional colleagues and by health authorities and trusts—its 'corporate identity'. Could the team make their identity and their mission explicit, both within and outside the organization—for example by an annual report?

Puzzles or problems?

'The puzzle is an embarrassment to which a solution already exists, although it may be hard to find even for the most accomplished of experts'.   (Revans 1986)

Common examples are the crossword puzzle, the end game at chess, and the geometrical examination question. Many medical decisions can be categorized as puzzles, for which there is a solution, if only we, or another expert, can find it. Much of general practice is like this. The patient may be suffering from a disease which has to be diagnosed and treated correctly, according to established norms, if such exist. If they do not exist, then treatment is a problem.

The problem, on the other hand, has no existing solution, and even after it has been long and deliberately treated by different persons, all skilled and reasonable, it may still suggest to each of them some different course of subsequent action. This will vary from one to another, in accordance with the differences between their past experiences, their current values and their future hopes.   (Revans 1986)

Problems, as stated above, may have no clear solution. They involve many alternatives and many imponderable factors, for example, should team members try to get neglected children taken into care? Should doctors exert pressure on their patients to have investigative or preventive procedures which they find distasteful? At what point should an elderly person be advised to give up their home and go into long-stay care? These problems may contain puzzles, but they involve a broad range of knowledge, experience, priorities, attitudes and values. For one professional group, like general practitioners or geriatricians, to be the arbiters and repository of society's ethical values, imposes an impossible burden upon them.

Teamwork allows a broader base of attitudes and values to be brought into the decision-making process. Each professional may have to think more deeply about a problem, but the decision can be shared. This was earlier quoted as an essential characteristic of teamwork, namely 'the team works by pooling knowledge, skills and resources and all members share responsibility for outcome'. As medicine becomes increasingly involved in caring for whole populations and the diseases affected by lifestyle and health beliefs, then team members can all expect to spend more time on problems, with less time left for the puzzles for which they were trained.

But health depends on knowledge and skills from outside medicine, and these may be contributed by a social worker. They are accustomed to dealing with problems that have no solution, in a context of uncertainty. This can contribute to the rich diversity of teamwork, but it may lead to misunderstandings arising from different views of the same bit of the world.

Decision making

What is an effective decision?

1. An effective decision must support the overall goals and values of the organization.

2. It must be logically sound, based on the best available information—but because logic is only infallible in retrospect, the decision must, at the time, **feel** like the right thing to do.

3. It must be acceptable to those who have to carry it out or abide by the results of the decision. For this to happen, those concerned must be involved from an early stage.

4. Its implementation and its likely success in meeting the original problem must be noted.

5. After implementation, any remaining problems or ill-effects must be sought out and information presented for a new decision. The process is thus a cycle, very similar to the management cycle.

A question that may arise is 'If it is such a good idea, why have we not done it already?' Perhaps there are positive by-products of staying as we are. How can we reach a solution which takes these into account and gives us the best of both worlds?

For decisions to be effective, they must be accepted and acted upon. This can be seen as having five stages:

- We **think** that it is a good idea;
- We **feel** that it is a good idea;
- We **decide** to do it;
- We **act**;
- We **confirm** that the decision has been carried out and has had the desired effects.

Avoiding pitfalls in decision making

Plovnick *et al.* (1978) quoted four main barriers to ideal decision making which can be used as a check-list:

1. Are we clear about, and agree on **what decision** we are trying to make?
2. Are we sure **who should be involved**, and have they been involved?
3. Are we sure **how people should be involved**, for example to provide information, to carry out the task, or to be the prime decision maker?
4. Are we sure about **the timing** of the decision, of its implementation or its monitoring? How urgent is it?

Implementation targets

When an important decision is taken, a note must be made of who will be responsible for implementation, and a series of targets defined. These can cover the dates when various stages of the project are to be completed and the interval before the outcome is reviewed. Someone must be nominated to keep an eye on the targets in case people forget. A wall planner may be useful for representing targets graphically.

Managing self-time and team time

Time is a critical factor in teamwork. People have to be motivated to 'find' or 'make' time. They need to turn up punctually at meetings. If a doctor is fifteen minutes late for a meeting of eight people, then two hours of valuable time has been wasted, quite apart from the anger that has been generated which may spill over into the meeting or into subsequent activity. Keeping meetings small (as for functional teams) helps to motivate people to be punctual. Punctuality is such an important virtue in teamwork, because of its 'multiplier' effect, that it needs to become part of team 'custom and practice' to keep to time. Emergencies can be cited as excuses, but they are infrequent, and why do some people seem to have all the emergencies? Understanding the nature and value of other people's time should be an essential part of health care, of teamwork, and indeed of everyday life. We talk of empathy in the consultation. 'Time empathy' describes this sensitivity to other people's perceptions of time (Pritchard 1992).

Different team members may operate on a different scale of urgency: doctors are often 'people in a hurry'. Some professionals may have less of a 'do it now—in five minutes it may be too late' style of working. Yet they may get angry with—for example—social workers who do not respond instantly to suspected cases of child abuse. Huntington (1981b) has characterized GPs as having a different time orientation to other members of the team, because of their greater preoccupation with pressure of time. Unless these underlying issues are understood and taken into account, tempers may well get frayed. If a professional cannot manage time effectively, work and domestic life will suffer, and the result may be workaholism and burnout. This process may be more obvious to team members than to the sufferer, and this presents an opportunity for the team to exercise its supportive role.

A check-list on managing self and time appears below:

MANAGING ONESELF

What am I here for? What are my values and purpose?

Make a list of what you have to do and categorize your tasks into **active positive tasks**—those you must do to achieve your purpose—the primary objectives of your work; and **reactive tasks**—those that land on your desk every day, that must be done to keep things moving.

Priorities must be established in the light of the importance and urgency of your tasks

Before you can time-schedule your tasks, you need to know **how long** you want to spend on each (this will reflect its importance: the closer the relationship of the task to 'what I'm here for', the greater its importance); and how soon you have to get it done (its urgency).

Importance and urgency are not the same thing

Then you must **schedule your time** for dealing with active positive tasks (or they won't get done). Then **allow time** for reactive tasks.

If a task is urgent and important, then do it now and spend time on it. If the task is urgent but not important, do it soon and do it quickly. If it is important but not urgent, then allocate time before it becomes urgent. If the task is neither urgent nor important, then you can postpone action, but leave it on the list.

With acknowledgement to *The unorganized manager*, Video Arts Ltd

Procedures—communication

Much of this section has been concerned with procedures, but two linked topics will be discussed in more detail, namely communication and meetings. The strength of working in a small team from the same building is that people meet every day or several times a day. The opportunities to exchange information, make decisions, and to socialize are numerous. Some formality can be introduced, by having regular lunch-time meetings, or letting it be known that people can 'catch the doctor during the coffee break'. Again, some time-discipline is needed, or people have a long wait or fail to meet, so a back-up system is needed.

Communication is a two-way process, and the first stage is to **listen**. When communication is one way, for example in a leaflet or questionnaire, we need to ensure that we first listen to the recipients when wording them, and give an opportunity for discussion later if possible. Likewise in the team, unless we listen to other people, no one will listen to us.

For procedures to 'stick' they must be simple, essential and natural.

Messages

Patients' lives and well-being may depend on the efficient passing of messages. Many methods are in use, from small written messages (sometimes using printed memo forms so that date and time are noted), to a daybook which everyone uses as an ingrained habit. Some general practices have a 'death book' in which the date and name of all practice patients who have died is entered as promptly as possible. Someone, such as the senior receptionist or secretary, has to have a monitoring role, so that urgent messages are passed immediately, and no messages are left in the air. Similarly with messages from patients, there must be a clear system of recording who they are for, and whether their receipt has been acknowledged by the recipient. When telephone or personal contact is difficult, then a personal facsimile machine or electronic mail can be very convenient. Communication is the life blood of team working, and without an efficient system there will be frustration and lack of trust.

Running effective meetings

All team meetings follow the pattern of group interaction, and the guidelines are clear, but rarely observed. Taking the chair is the focus, and this is considered later, but a lot can be done before and after meetings to ensure their success. Much of this work can be done by the practice manager or unit secretary in consultation with the chair. The following hints have been clearly set out in the Video Arts booklets and training films (starring John Cleese) *Meetings, bloody meetings* and *More bloody meetings*, which are strongly recommended for educating and entertaining team members (see p. 135).

Planning ahead: What is the meeting trying to achieve? Think through the objectives.

Pre-notification: Tell those who are coming to the meeting what is to be discussed and why—concisely and in good time.

Preparation: The agenda must be in proper sequence, when one decision affects another. Time must be allocated and rationed according to the importance of the subject.

Processing: Discussion of each item needs some structure, so that people do not stray from the point, repeat themselves, or indulge in private conversation.
Whoever takes the chair must understand group behaviour and ensure that any conflict is creative rather than destructive.

Putting it on record: A clear summary of events, decisions made, and action to be taken and by whom.

Many team meetings occur at lunch-time. The manager or secretary must ensure that all potential attenders know the date and time of the meeting, and what is to be discussed. Members should be reminded of the meeting a few days ahead if it is important.

Business meetings run better if they are properly set up, with tables for papers, and seats in a circle or square, so all can see the chairperson and each other. Any reference books or information should be available. The manager or secretary will have to consider what questions might be asked, and have the answers ready. Everyone must know how much time is allotted to each item so that the business will be completed before people start to drift away. Great skill will be needed to complete the business of the meeting without stifling discussion, otherwise some people will not feel committed to the decision, and so will not implement it willingly. The practice manager or secretary must work closely with the chair and brief him or her for the meeting. Someone will need to take the minutes and circulate them.

For further study of meetings, material is available from Video Arts as videos and booklets which are listed on p. 135. Some of these may be available from the training department of the local Health Authority.

Learning exercise 5: Ways of getting things done

Aim: To explore the communication and decision-making processes within the team.

Objectives: By the end of the session participants will have:

(1) read the relevant recommended reading and completed issues cards.
(2) become aware of the priority issues facing the team.
(3) developed a list of priorities of issues for the team.
(4) begun to develop an action plan to tackle the issues.

What are the most important issues for the team?

If necessary, allow 10 minutes for reading Section 5 and write down on a card what you think are the most important issues facing the team (up to three), and hand them in for collation. Refer back to Section 3 to ensure that the issues are relevant to key goals. The leader should present the collated responses in the order of frequency of mention.

As an alternative, the issues can be written on 'post-it' notes and then 'clustered' to help find groups of related issues.

What are the priorities for individuals and for the team? (See check-list on p. 62.) Agree the top priority item and start to develop an action plan if time allows. Further action planning could be carried out as a sub-project.

Facilitator summary

Materials: Completed 'issues' cards, flip-chart paper, 'post-it' notes.

Activity: Revision of recommended reading (10 min)

Completion of 'issues' cards

Collation of issues. Ensure these are relevant to key goals (as stated in Session 4)

Present the responses in order of frequency of mention (10 min).

With participants, list items in order of priority on flip-chart paper.

Agree top priority. Ask group to start an action plan on this priority (4 min).

Optional (needs extra time). Other issues in order of priority can be addressed at other specially arranged times.

For the next meeting

Please read Section 6 (pp. 68–72), and write down on one side of a card (which will not be collected), what you see as the five most important attributes of a leader. It may be helpful to classify these under the headings of: (1) personal qualities and beliefs, (2) skills, and (3) working practices (but not more than five in total).

Secondly, please consider in what aspects of your own working life you need to show leadership. This could be written on the back of the card. Please bring the card to the next meeting.

Section 6: Team leadership

Leaders may appear because they have vision, ideas, energy, persuasiveness, and make the right decisions; but mostly because they are trusted. Leadership is not a matter of clever manipulation of others, but more of having the capability to provide the best solutions at the right moment, which others feel they can accept. In a team, the person who is committed to carrying out most of the task, particularly the difficult bits, may become the leader for that task.

Are leaders born or made? Some people seem to be natural leaders, but those who are not can learn to lead. We are all faced with situations in which we have to lead, so how can we refine our skills as leaders? In a primary health care or specialist team, a doctor has the opportunity to be the accepted leader for much of the time, but only if he or she has the talent for it. Leadership must be learned and earned: it cannot be taken for granted.

Leadership qualities

What are the personal qualities that encourage people to accept a leader? Some are listed below. An effective leader:

- inspires trust;
- is a good listener;
- selects good staff;
- has infectious enthusiasm;
- runs effective meetings;
- speaks and presents information well;
- accepts responsibility;
- is calm under stress;
- can tolerate uncertainty;
- responds positively to conflict and failure;

- helps people to see the funny side of things;

- has a ready smile.

The work that general practitioners do in the consultation, as described by Byrne and Long (1976), has the same characteristics that were called leadership by earlier writers on management. So general practitioners, equally with specialists, are likely to have considerable experience and skill in leading patients back to health, but can these skills be applied in leading an organization like a team, and can these qualities be enhanced? There is good evidence that doctors can improve their skills in the consultation by training and assessment (Pendleton *et al.* 1984). So too should they be able to enhance the parallel skills of leadership. Self-assessment and peer-assessment are the keys to improving skills in the consultation, but what measures of leadership skill can be used?

Who leads the team?

Members of the team from other professions have similar skills. So who leads the team, and is it always the same person? By tradition the senior doctor is cast in the role of leader. This may not work very well in the doctors' (functional) team where the younger ones may want change and the older ones have little motivation to alter the *status quo*. In the health care teams, with their wide range of disciplines, the question of leadership must be addressed afresh. Changing situations may need different kinds of leader, and some tasks may be better led by someone other than the usual team leader. Doctors might try an experiment with rotating leadership in their own team, and see how it works— some already do this, and find that different aspects of the work need different leaders.

Kinds of leadership

Natural leaders have many ways of leading. Different situations demand different styles. When the building is on fire, the leader does not call a meeting! But when there is a delicate staff problem, a more listening and reflective approach pays off. Leadership behaviour occupies a spectrum, between the extremes of 'boss-centred leadership' and 'subordinate-centred leadership', with many shades of behaviour in between. Effective leaders should be able to vary their way of leading according to the situation.

Some leaders are 'charismatic' in that they have special (super-human?) qualities that set them apart from the rest. They lead and everyone follows, often uncritically. Charisma has its uses, but it is no substitute for sensitive and flexible team leadership that is uniquely suited to the people, the situation, and the tasks. 'Inspirational' leadership is another matter, whereby a leader infects others with the enthusiasm to achieve shared goals. Another categorization of leadership describes three styles—the author-itarian or 'tells' style, the consulting or 'listening-questioning' style, and a further style of *laissez faire* or non-leadership. Alas, this third style can happen in general and hospital practice when the potential leaders have become overwhelmed by workload and 'burnt out'. Often they are very conscientious, but do not have the capability to manage time and workload. They may still hold on to the authority of their position, but by failing to fulfil their leadership role, they end up with no power in an ineffective organization. These three styles of leadership are described below:

Authoritarian

The authoritarian or 'tells' style of leadership is characterized by all the decision making and planning being concentrated in the leader, so that there is no encouragement of creative thinking or open discussion. Work is allocated from above. People's work is taken for granted, with consequent low job satisfaction.

Consulting

The consulting or 'listening–questioning' style is characterized by a leader who is approachable, and who involves the staff in decisions and discusses problems. Work allocation is left more to the staff, and creative thinking is encouraged. People feel valued, job satisfaction and morale tend to be high, and work gets done well and effectively.

Laissez-faire

The *laissez-faire* style is characterized by inconsistent and irresponsible leadership. The leader cannot be pinned down, and is not trusted. Staff have to fend for themselves, and tend to choose their own leader. Morale is low, and the work does not get done.

Shared leadership

By focusing on the goal and the task, teamwork becomes more manageable. If the task particularly concerns one team member, he or she can exercise leadership in that task, with support from the team and without any threat to the usual leader. In this way, many tense situations can be defused and the teamwork can proceed smoothly. By spreading the leadership around the team, each member can feel a greater sense of responsibility and fulfilment. To take an analogy from football. Off the field, the manager's word may rule, but once the game starts, leadership passes to the person who has the ball.

In health care, much of the decision making takes place when the professional is alone, or with the patient. In this way each professional is a leader, but who leads the team? We have already questioned whether it should necessarily be the senior doctor? Does it have to be the same person all the time? The message of this workbook is that leadership is earned by the ability to weld the diverse talents and activities of the team into effective patient care, not just assumed because of age or status. In the case of a housebound patient with chronic illness, the patient or the carer may, in effect, lead the intrinsic team.

Further information about running meetings is available in Locke, M. (1980). *How to run committees and meetings*. London, Papermac. Also in Pemberton, M. (1982). *Guide to effective meetings*. The Industrial Society (see address on p. 134).

Learning exercise 6: Exploring the nature of leadership

This exercise is a group discussion of attributes of leaders, occasions when each team member has to lead and whether any training for leadership is needed.

Aim: To explore the nature of leadership.

Objectives: By the end of the session participants will have:

(1) read the relevant recommended reading;

(2) listed what they consider the five most important attributes of a leader;

(3) listed the aspects of their life in which they need to show leadership;

(4) produced a list representing the consensus of the group on leadership qualities;

(5) discussed the adequacy of leadership in their own role;

(6) **Optional**—defined the needs for any further leadership training.

Form into 'single discipline' groups of not more than five people. If necessary, allow ten minutes to read Section 6, and list individually:

(1) what you consider to be the five most important attributes of a leader?

and

(2) in what aspects of your working life you need to show leadership?

Compare your lists of the attributes of leadership with those of others in your group, and produce a list representing your combined views. Then discuss in your own group:

(1) the part played by leadership in your own role;

(2) whether you feel that further training is needed; and

(3) what this training should aim to achieve.

After 30 minutes, re-form the main group and discuss the conclusions of the sub-groups. One team member should keep a record of any conclusions. If further development of leadership is requested, this could be set up as a sub-project, either 'in-house' or as an outside training course. Decide what future action is needed.

Facilitator summary

Materials: *Flip-chart paper, individual cards*

Activities: *Revise recommended reading (10 min).*

Ask participants to form into single discipline groups and to list individually:

(i) *What they consider to be the five most important attributes of a leader.*

(ii) *In what aspects of their working life they need to show leadership (10 min).*

Ask each group to:

(i) *Compare their lists of attributes and to produce a common list (20 min).*

(ii) *(a) Discuss the part played by leadership in their own role;*

(b) *State whether they feel further training is needed;*

(c) *State what further training should aim toachieve.*

Re-form the main group. Discuss the main conclusions of the sub-group. Ask someone to keep a note of comments (20 min).

Optional *(requires more time). Ask how leadership could be further developed.*

For the next meeting

Please read Section 7 (pp. 76–8). Then imagine:

(1) *first* that you have just joined the team, and
(2) *then* that you are about to leave the group and your successor has just been appointed.

Then fill in the questionnaire below, on four separate cards numbered 1–4 and bring them (unsigned) to the next meeting. The information on the cards is to be shared.

QUESTIONNAIRE FOR SESSION 7

Please fill in on four numbered cards your answers to the following questions.

1. Think back to when you were new to the team

Card 1. 'What should I have told the team about myself?'

Card 2. 'What questions should I have asked of other team members?

2. A successor has just been appointed as you are leaving

Card 3. 'What questions should the team members ask the new appointee?'

Card 4. 'What should team members tell the new appointee?'

Section 7: New team members

A really effective and contented team, with the highest possible standards and morale is a very formidable prospect for the newcomer (or even for the established team member whose visits are infrequent). Though they may soon pick up the feeling that 'this is a nice place to work', they feel daunted by the way everyone knows what to do and they do not. Sometimes they may have to work on their own and not know when or who to ask. What can be done to help them to settle in, so that they feel that they are a competent and valued member of the team?

'Sitting by Nellie' is not enough. The newcomer can observe how Nellie behaves, but not why she does one thing rather than another. When questioned, Nellie, if she is a real expert, may not be able to explain. So some induction training is helpful, and this is certainly the message from industry.

The difficulty that a new member experiences in joining a team will depend a lot on how they came to join. Entrants may be new employees, or members of health or social work professions attached to the team. In the case of a new receptionist, have they been carefully selected and briefed so that they know what is expected of them? Do the employers know of their skills and experience and possible gaps to be filled by training? Professional staff such as practice nurses, would need to discuss individual training needs with doctors and colleagues, who would all benefit if the training is provided.

A new staff member will have been appointed by people outside the team. But was a team member invited to meet the candidates, or even (as a privilege) to sit in on the appointment committee as an observer? Should doctors not reciprocate by inviting other team members to participate in the appointment of a new team member?

Does the new appointee really want to join the team? What has been their experience of teamwork in previous posts? Have they had a chance to visit the premises and meet all the staff? Even if all these obstacles have been overcome, there are many more. Successful teamwork depends on mutual trust, and this means that people can predict how their team colleagues will behave in specific circumstances. For example, a doctor may persuade a patient to see a social worker, but what if the social worker does not regard the referral as appropriate? Is this mismatch of expectations and reality approached in the spirit of learning or of rejection?

Induction training of a new employee or team member

Ellis (1984, 1990) spelled out the messages very clearly for general practice, but the message is a general one. His work is worth reading before a new employee is even recruited. He emphasized that well-trained and competent staff are worth their weight in gold. Not only do they make life easier for doctors and patients, but their adequate induction and training is a responsibility of the partners for which they might be held legally liable. In hospital teams the process is likely to be more remote, but close consultation with the personnel officer and members of the appointing committee may save expensive mistakes.

From the employees' viewpoint, they may have started the job with high hopes, only to find that no one helps them in the way that they need. So a first step, as in all learning, is to discover the learning needs. This would normally be a job for the practice or unit manager, but all the staff may need to play a part. Hence the problems should be discussed in a team meeting before the new employee arrives, and the learning process, and the employee's morale closely monitored.

In the case of attached staff, training is the responsibility of their managers, and indeed they are sometimes trained in how to make the most of teamwork. But informal training for working in the new team can only be done 'in-house', using a project such as this. The extent to which existing team members are prepared to invest in training new appointees will be a measure of the cohesion of the team. It is no surprise that where attached staff are not made to feel welcome, their primary loyalties are to their own discipline, who may work as an area team that is separate from the practice. Learning local rules—particularly the informal ones—will be helped if they are explicit and agreed, so that the messages are not contradictory. The more there is in writing the better, provided that the rules or guidelines are clear, and do really represent current 'custom and practice', not just a shedding of responsibility.

This training takes time and forethought. The unit manager must not throw the new employee in at the deep end, but allow time for familiarization and learning, using a mutually agreed programme. All health care staff work under very great pressure, and if this is a new experience, a lot of help will be needed in order to adapt. All team members can do their bit by seeing that the new employee is settling in well, and has a clear view of the goals of the team and of the values that underpin the work of the team.

So far, we have assumed that the employee has come from outside, but induction problems may also arise when someone is promoted to a new role within the team (for example from senior secretary to practice manager). An outside training course may be a useful expedient.

Fitting in to teamwork

Given the complexity of tasks, roles, procedures and relation-ships, any new entrant will find that it takes time to get the feel of the new team. It will indeed be a new team each time someone joins, requiring a mutual learning process. For all that the new entrant will have a lot to learn, so will the other team members need to discover the skills and potential contribution of the new-comer. Some of the exercises in this booklet, such as the 'diagnostic instrument' in Section 2 could be tried once more.

Learning exercise 7: Information transfer

This exercise deals with matching new members' expectations to the team's norms, and producing a manual, or guidelines for new staff.

Aim: To produce guidelines for new staff that communicate the team's norms.

Objectives: By the end of the session participants will have:

(1) read the relevant recommended reading and have completed the questionnaire.

(2) discussed the answers from the questionnaire.

(3) **Optional**—collated the information into a brief guide for new team members.

If necessary, allow ten minutes to read Section 7, and complete the four cards as shown (p. 75).

For the first question, take turns to read out your answers. What are the common themes? Go round the group again for each subsequent question. If time allows, or as a sub-project, collate the information into a brief guide for new team members. If there is a newly-joined team member, he or she might like to help with the booklet.

Facilitator summary

Materials: *Flip-chart paper, completed cards (4)*
Activity: *Revise recommended reading and complete the four cards(10 min).*

Ask participants to read out their answers.

Summarize these on flip-chart paper and highlight common themes. Do this for subsequent questions (50 min).

> **Optional** *(needs further time). Suggest to the group that they collate the information into a brief guide for new team members.*

For the next meeting

Please read Section 8, and complete one more section of a team diagnostic questionnaire as set out below (as on pp. 25–31, Section 2). This should be completed in good time and handed (unsigned) to the collator, who should complete a further team diagnostic summary, and bring it to the next meeting along with the original summary sheet from Section 2.

In addition, please answer the question 'What single change in the way we work would have the greatest effect on improving my morale?' Write down the answer on a card and bring it to the next session (not for collection).

CONFIDENTIAL QUESTIONNAIRE ON
TEAM WORKING—PART 2

4. What it feels like to work in this team (*cont.*)

Feeling of value
Please read both statements, and ring one letter which seems closest to the way your team functions:

Statement I 'I often feel that some team members do not think that other team members have much of a contribution to make. I do not personally get the feeling that my contribution is valued by other team members'.

    a. Just like statement I
    b. More like I than II
    c. In between I and II
    d. More like II than I
    e. Just like statement II

Statement II 'Everyone recognizes that the work would not get done without everyone giving of their best. Each member of the team, including myself, is treated as an important part of the team. It gives the feeling that you and your job are important and valued'.

Examples:

....

....

Section 8: Working in a team

How does it feel to work in this team?

This topic was the focus of four questions in the 'diagnostic instrument' undertaken earlier in the programme. The questions covered participation in teamwork, managing conflict, availability to each other and mutual support. The original instrument (Plovnick *et al.* 1978) contained another topic about the recognition of the contribution that people were making. This is part of the practical exercise below.

Availability

Communicating is an effort, and if someone is never available when wanted, or the telephone is always engaged or goes unanswered, or once contacted they have no time to spare, then people give up. Doctors may play 'hard to get', as they have the image of being busy people, and they do not like to be disturbed during a consultation. If the morning break is the time to meet and communicate, they may often run late. Can people who are hard to contact, expect others to be easily available? Can we achieve a balance, so that communication is effective?

Mutual support

Teamwork, by its very nature, includes the sharing of responsibility. If we all go along with a decision and the outcome is a failure, then we all bear some responsibility for it, even if ours was not the deed that preceded the failure. Conversely, a successful outcome is good for everyone's morale and we can all share the satisfaction. In all areas of health care, where staff and patients all have their share of human frailty, where uncertainty is the norm and everyone dies eventually, failure is frequent but still hard to bear. If team members, as individuals, are deeply committed to their work, they are bound to suffer when their patients suffer. Team members, when meeting as a group that trusts one another, can detach themselves a little from the sadness that surrounds them, and give each other this support. Just to recognize each other's suffering goes a long way to healing it. Some more practical help can be worked out, whereby team members can take turn about with breaking bad news and support of the terminally ill and bereaved. They can also try to find a moment to discuss their feelings of grief or failure.

When team members, who have outside managers, are having their professional autonomy curtailed, or their contribution to the team threatened in other ways, those managers must realize that they are damaging teamwork and may be taking on the whole team. A well-integrated team that has clear goals has, often un-realized, authority and power.

Recognition of the value of everyone's contribution

A basic tenet of teamwork, is that everyone is doing as well as they can, and that the value of their contribution is appreciated. For this to happen, each team member must be prepared to tell the others how much their work is valued. Everyone has times when they feel the effort is too great and the benefits too small. On these occasions, a colleague's word or gesture of appreciation brings out the sun again. This does not mean that a team is an uncritical 'mutual admiration society', but that in the setting of a team, people are aware of their own value, and should be keen to recognize the qualities of their (equally valued) colleagues.

Appreciation of each other's value is a basic motivating factor in group behaviour, and an essential ingredient of morale. The message in this paragraph is, perhaps, the single most important one in this workbook and cannot be repeated too often.

Job satisfaction

A feeling that all the effort is worthwhile, that this is a good place to work, that colleagues are liked and trusted, that people know where they are heading—all these make for job satisfaction. Team members can all expect to have a feeling of pleasure for a job well done. Pay and conditions, security of employment and staff appraisal are all important too, but are never enough on their own to keep people happy at work. Perhaps a better word is morale, and that is the next topic.

Morale in the team

An important indicator of the state of health of an organization is its morale ('conduct and behaviour with regard to confidence, hope, zeal, etc.' *Oxford English Dictionary*). Morale is an intangible quality of an individual or an organization which not only measures the success of their efforts, but also potentiates that success. If morale is high, setbacks can be overcome without depressing the functioning of the individual or group. Morale includes adaptability, confidence, and hope—a feeling that things will come out right in the end. It is a corporate feeling of the power to win through, whatever the obstacles.

One factor that harms morale is uncertainty about the future. This is the price that is paid for any fundamental organizational change imposed from above, such as have been experienced in the UK with successive reorganizations of the NHS since 1974. But morale—of a sort—may also be high in a profession that is too secure and over-confident and insensitive to consumer needs. So high morale needs to walk a tightrope. But if team members keep close to patients and sensitive to their needs, then the tightrope is nearer the ground and less threatening. Working in a team helps this closeness and confidence.

A balance sheet might be drawn up of factors favouring high morale in an individual or an organization, and those factors that tend to lower morale. Each of us can draw up our own list. This is an example:

These factors may be helpful to morale:

- a small organization that communicates well;
- high quality and level of training of staff;

- high motivation and dedication;
- clear sense of direction and goals shared by all;
- organizational stability—low staff turnover;
- sensitivity to patients' needs;
- quality assurance with results shared with all concerned;
- regular reports of progress towards goals and targets;
- an open style of organization and leadership;
- adaptability to change;
- able to contain conflict or use it constructively.

Many of these factors reinforce each other. The factors that harm morale are the obverse of those listed, and they too can reinforce each other. In this way a vicious spiral of inefficiency, poor quality of care, and decreasing morale can set in which requires heroic methods of rescue on all fronts. The team diagnostic instrument reflects the team's state of morale, and this topic will be addressed in Learning exercise 8.

Conflict in the team

Conflict, as mentioned earlier, is the very stuff of human interaction, and to avoid it entirely would be difficult and probably harmful. Indeed, conflict that is handled openly, and takes account of team members' individuality, can deepen mutual understanding and respect. Conflicts often appear as a clash of personalities, but may really represent a conflict of values and beliefs. If these can be explored and understood, the result may be a diversion of energy from conflict into creativity.

Conflicts can, however, get out of hand, or develop a life of their own, and so distract people from more pressing tasks. So how do conflicts arise and how can we contain them, or even make them useful? Huntington (1981a) has made a particular study of conflict in primary health teams, but its message is universal.

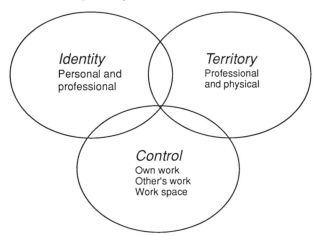

Fig. 7. Huntington's triad of determinants of conflict.

She identified three underlying areas in which conflict might arise, as shown in Fig. 7.

Identity   This covers one's personal identity including self-image, self respect, and the sort of person we perceive ourselves to be. Professional identity describes how we see ourselves in the job—as a nurse, doctor, secretary, etc. Professional identity is tied up with the status and respect given by society to a profession, and the clarity of the professional role, as seen by other professionals and the public. New, or rapidly changing professions may be very uncertain of their role. This is important within the team. Doctors enjoy high public esteem; they are the most highly paid members of the team; their role is now fairly clear to themselves and the public (though undergoing change at the moment). The profession, like nursing, is an old and stable one. Social workers and health visitors, by contrast, have considerable role uncertainty and may get a bad press. Their pay is low in relation to their long training and heavy load of responsibility. Professionals need to feel that the public and team members value what they do, but they also need to have a strong sense of personal value. These feelings should be perceived equally by the lay members of staff, who must not be devalued because of their lack of professional status.

Territory   This can be professional territory—that is the extent of each person's job, or it can be physical—in terms of room and desk space, and where we keep our belongings. Professional territory corresponds to our role, and squabbles are more likely to occur at the boundaries, where our role might impinge on someone else's. Or there may be gaps between roles, so that there are some jobs that nobody wants to do.

Physical territory, or space is often a source of conflict, but as Huntington (1981a) pointed out, what seems like a conflict over space, for example where the new computer or a noisy printer is sited, may really be about professional identity and status. The people of low status may get pushed around, and this is a function of power.

Attached nursing staff working in a health centre may have their 'own' suite of rooms, over which they exercise day-to-day control. However, in a surgery or medical centre in which they have an office, they may not feel the same territorial security, and conflicts may arise over use of shared space. In hospital, 'ownership' of space is very insecure.

Control   This is all about power, and whose wants take precedence, as in a pecking order of chickens or a hierarchical organization. Delegation of tasks tends to be from the powerful to those of less power, as is the giving and accepting of orders, and the allocation of time. Doctors may feel that they have an overriding legal responsibility for their patients, but other professionals feel that they have similar responsibilities. Lay staff are usually highly motivated, so their responsibility is moral rather than legal. But it is responsibility none the less. To support this sense of responsibility, everyone must have control over a part of their work and work environment. Without it their role is diminished and their identity shrinks to a shadow.

Interaction of the three determinants

The message of Huntington's triad of identity, territory and control is that every conflict can be seen in terms of all three, and we need to look very closely at all three factors, as the obvious one may not be the real cause of the conflict, and they all interact. Similarly, when planning changes, they can be assessed in terms of all three factors for possible good and ill effects. Members of an effective and contented team have come to terms with the issues of their own and their colleagues' personal and professional identity, their professional and physical territory, and everyone's need for control over some of their work and working environment.

Some varieties of dysfunction

Ways that team working can go wrong have already been mentioned. A team member may be reluctant to fill in a questionnaire or to join in a discussion. Should they be asked for their views during a meeting, or just given an opportunity to join in if they want? Full team meetings can be disrupted by people who enjoy being provocative, or by two people who are mutually antagonistic and carry on their private battles in front of the team. A leader may want to keep the business of the meeting going, or may prefer to bring the conflict out into the open for discussion.

Methods already described, such as role negotiation and role messages, may help (see Section 4), or exploring the issues in terms of identity, territory, and control. Sometimes these attempts to heal have the opposite effect, and reveal the deep nature of the conflict, and so provoke one of the team members to withdraw from teamwork or leave. Should the other team members try to prevent this 'divorce', encourage it, or keep out of the conflict? There are no certain rules, any more than there are for marriage guidance, but outside help may be useful.

Severe conflict—is outside help needed?

Some teams are riven by conflict, or as a result of past conflict, may keep communication to a minimum. As a consequence, team members keep to their own domain behind the barriers of misunderstanding or firmly entrenched attitudes. An important theme of this book is that by focusing on goals and tasks and then on roles and procedures, people will have the confidence to come out of their trenches, and destructive conflict will be minimized. But when conflict is severe, it may be difficult to get the team development going, or even ensure a minimal level of day-to-day teamwork without outside help (see Introduction, p. 5).

Just as when we are ill, we do our best to get better with our own resources. When that is not enough, we seek professional help. So with the team, we should be prepared to call in outside help from someone with suitable skill and experience. Some health authorities employ 'organization development' consultants and 'facilitators', or will contribute part of the cost. A list of organizations and individuals who might help appears on p. 136.

Different consultants would approach the team's problems in different ways. One common method is for the consultant to have interviews in confidence with all the staff, in order to get a general picture of the team and a 'diagnosis' of what is amiss. Then a series of group sessions would be held with team members, or the whole team, and the 'healing' process would be started. There are advantages in using someone independent of the team. Group and plenary meetings can be arranged at an outside venue, like a retreat, with time for reflection as well as group work. This method is widely used by industry, but is more costly. They regard it as a worthwhile investment of time and money.

Methods such as role-play and conceptual modelling have not been mentioned so far, as they might need skills that all teams do not possess. Facilitators might like to apply them (see Sections 13 and 14). However, those teams who have experience of these methods, might like to try them where appropriate, or invite a facilitator to help.

Learning exercise 8: Team feelings

In this exercise we apply one more section of the 'diagnostic instrument' about feeling valued in the team and discuss the results. Ways of raising morale are identified, and plans made for doing so.

Aim: To explore individual feelings about team membership and ways to increase morale.

Objectives: By the end of the session participants will have:

(1) read the relevant recommended reading and completed the questionnaire;

(2) discussed issues arising from the results of this questionnaire, in comparison to the previous one;

(3) identified what single change to the way of working would have greatest effect on improving individual morale;

(4) produced an action plan on what is discovered in (3);

(5) **Optional**—made a plan of action to improve morale based on the results of discussion by everyone.

If necessary, allow 10 minutes to read Section 8, complete a further diagnostic questionnaire, and write down the answer to the question:

'What single change to the way we work that would have the greatest effect on improving my morale?'

The collator should have completed the summary sheet for the additional question about feeling valued as a team member. The results can be shown to the full group and compared with the earlier summary sheet. What issues arise for the team? (20 min).

Working in groups of three (of different disciplines), consider the changes in working practices that most affect members' morale, and see what consensus can be reached and action planned (20 min).

Re-form the full group to hear reports from the small groups and make plans for action. One team member could lead a sub-project to take action on other issues raised.

Facilitator summary

Materials: Completed final part of team diagnostic questionnaire;
answer to question on card, completed diagnostic summary sheet.

Activity: Revise recommended reading and answer the question:
'What single change to the way we work would have the greatest effect on improving my morale?' (10 min).

Share results of completed diagnostic summary sheet.
Compare this with results of earlier summary sheet (as used in Session 3) (10 min).

Ask participants to split into multidiscipline sets. Ask them to consider what changes in working practices most affect their morale (20 min).

Encourage reaching an agreement, and ordering priorities. Then ask for action plan on top priority (20 min).

Optional (requires extra time). Reconvene whole group. Summarize any other issues. Produce action plans for dealing with these.

For the next meeting

We will be discussing the world outside the team, so please read Section 9, and prepare a list of the people or organizations outside the team to which you need to relate as part of your work, and consider the sort of links that are needed. Bring the list to the next meeting.

D The team environment

Section 9: The world outside the team—shared care

The team as an 'open system'

When locked in a 'hot' consultation with a difficult patient, the doctor may forget that there is a world outside, or even outside the consulting room. The boundary of the consulting room is the door and the telephone line, but what is the boundary of professional work or of the team? Other team professionals have the same issues to face; their boundaries are difficult to define. Are patients within the system, or in the outside world—or both? Likewise with other professionals and lay staff. They spend much of their day in the work setting, though many have outside commitments. But more of their time they spend in their homes and neighbourhoods and as part of their family.

The health care team as an organization or 'system' has a poorly defined boundary with the outside world, that is to say it is an 'open system' (Pritchard *et al.* 1984). Open systems are characterized by their being closely integrated with the world in which they operate. They contain people, working at tasks in a structure, and linked by many processes such as communication, cooperation and decision making. People, tasks, and structure are interdependent, so changing one inevitably alters the other, for example appointing new staff affects tasks and organizational structure.

An open system has an input of people with health problems, information and money and an output (one hopes) of improved health, and satisfied patients and staff. Input and output are linked by 'feedback' so that the system remains stable in spite of changes in demand, information, cash flow, and so on.

The health care team is a good example of an open system. Outside organizations are also open systems, and people outside the team, with whom one has to deal, are likely to be involved in the processes described above. So if we want to cooperate with someone with whom we deal, their own circumstances must be taken into account. So the first step in managing the outside world is to understand how one's own organization works and consider the workings of outside organizations as well.

Cooperating in shared (or integrated) care

When a patient is referred to a specialist by a general practitioner, responsibility for care is shared. If admitted to hospital, the specialist takes full responsibility. If treated and discharged from the hospital, the general practitioner is responsible. But between these extremes are many variants of 'shared care'. The patient (as in antenatal care or radiotherapy) may attend both sites and be cared for by both teams. In other conditions (such as diabetes), the patient may keep away from hospital, but the primary health care team receives support from the specialist team. This can be by telephone advice, technological support such as laboratory tests, and increasingly by 'telemedicine', where new technology allows the problem rather than the patient to make the journey. Examples are video-conferencing giving a simulated consultation, or telemetering of blood samples or ECGs. But the key agent is the facilitator or specialist nurse, with a foot in both camps, who can help with the transfer of knowledge, skills, and resources.

If we assume that 20 specialist departments might be involved (out of a total of 56 specialist categories in the UK) in shared care with 30 practices in a district, then 600 linkages are needed. This means that developing, say, a primary health care team and a diabetic specialist unit into a single team is not realistic. They must remain separate teams, linked by common aims, procedures, guidelines, and goodwill. The specific and very difficult problems of care shared between two teams will be considered in Sections 13 (tools for shared care) and 14 (the role of the facilitator).

Shared care is also at work within hospitals, between secondary and tertiary care, and between departments. The same principles and methods of cooperation can be applied, but the first step is to look at our own team and make sure it is functioning effectively. Shared care between poorly functioning teams has little chance of success.

Influencing organizations or people outside the team

It is tempting just to look after those parts of the organization that are under our control. But we are subject to outside influences, and should be able to exercise some influence outside our own team when this is thought to be beneficial. How do we go about 'active management' of the outside world? Is it possible? Or is it an interference in other people's affairs? Assuming that we have goals for our work and for our patients, many of them will involve people outside, and if we cannot influence them our patients will suffer. For example, if a doctor wishes that action is taken in a case of suspected child abuse, or a GP wishes to have an elderly person with abdominal pain admitted to hospital, they will have to influence other people or organizations, and bring them round to their way of thinking or seek some compromise. If a new building for the team is needed, many outside people must be persuaded to take action that suits everyone's needs.

Even for everyday matters, we need to operate in an organization that fits well into its environment, and is respected and well treated by people in other organizations. This means developing a climate of cooperation and goodwill in which people are keen to help us, because we have helped them, or because we can make out a convincing case for cooperation, or both.

Other people's viewpoints

Just as we have to understand the workings and complexity of our own organization, so we have to understand other people's viewpoints and problems, which we can only do if we have some knowledge of their problems and priorities, and how they view us. The better we can know key people personally and appreciate their viewpoint, the more easily will they understand ours.

So far the impression might be gained that if the team and relevant organizations and people are all one happy family, then our plans will go through, and our aspirations will be met. Life never was like that, as people's aims inevitably conflict, and some of the options for cooperation (for example attaching social workers to the general practice team) seem to be diminishing in the UK, in spite of an increasing need for such links. Whereas, in the past, it was possible to plan in a relatively stable environment, now the world outside is so turbulent, that we may need to abandon traditional planning, and just aim to survive until there is a lull in the storm.

Developing active networks

Links with the outside world need to be made and actively maintained. This will not happen on its own: someone must take the initiative. This may mean going to meet key people, inviting them to meetings—or better still to parties! In the case of patients, a patient advisory group might be considered (see next section).

Team members may need to draw up a list or map of all the people and organizations with whom links are needed, and check that these links are regularly reviewed to make sure that each sees the other's aims and role in a similar light. How often do people fail to cooperate because their goals are disparate or not articulated clearly, or the other's role is not clearly understood?

Learning exercise 9: Key people and organizations outside the team

Who are the key people and organizations to whom we have to relate? Compare lists of people and organizations outside the practice. Focus on a particular problem with an outside agency or person, and discuss ways of solving it.

Aim: To explore relationships with key people outside the team.

Objectives: By the end of the session participants will have:

(1) read the relevant recommended reading and prepared a list of people outside the team to whom they relate as part of their work;

(2) discussed the lists previously formed with particular reference to the sorts of links that need to be made;

(3) made an action plan to improve cooperation with one named outside team or organization;

(4) **Optional**—made action plans for other identified organizations.

If necessary, allow 5 minutes to read Section 9. All members will have been asked to bring a list of people or organizations with whom they have to relate as part of their work in the team.

Working in multidisciplinary groups of two to four, discuss the lists you have brought, and the sort of links that are needed (25 minutes).

Re-form the main group to hear from each of the small groups. Select one outside team or organization, in order to discuss issues and options for improving cooperation. Make action plans for this one group.

Plans for dealing with the people and organizations selected by the other team members can be made as a sub-project.

Facilitator summary

Materials: *List of 'outside' people and organizations*

Activity: *Revision of recommended reading (5 min), completion of lists*

Ask participants to separate into multidisciplinary sets and discuss the lists, identifying the sort of links needed (25 min).

Re-form the main group. Ask each group to report findings.

Selecting one outside organization, begin making action plans for improved communication and working with this group.

Optional *(more time needed). Other plans can be made for other organizations.*

For the next meeting

Please read Section 10 (pp. 99–101). Take the opportunity to ask several patients how they think services to patients might be improved, and write down their suggestions as below:

Card 1. Give up to three suggestions from patients for improving curative services.

Card 2. Give up to three suggestions from patients for improving preventative services.

Please bring the cards to the next meeting, for collection after the meeting.

Section 10: Patients as team members

Feedback from patients

The concept of the 'intrinsic team' inevitably involves the patient (and lay supporter) in teamwork at the individual level. But is this enough? Would it be helpful for involvement to occur also at the level of the team organization? In this way, the team as a whole could get some feedback about the quality and effectiveness of the care being provided.

The current trend in general practice is to pay more attention to the views of patients, for example when deciding on surgery times, the design of patient information leaflets, and screening forms and letters. Many practices make their annual report available to patients, but do not have any formal way of getting feedback. Some practices have a patient participation group involving nearly all the members of the team, though few now use that title. 'Health support group' or 'patient advisory group' sound much better. Where a group is in operation it does indeed support the practice with advice, skills and resources, and by doing so the members of the group hope to achieve better health and health care. Such a group could be regarded as a 'functional team' with responsibility for feedback and public relations. The episodic nature of much hospital work makes feedback from patients harder to achieve, but where it is in operation, it has been supportive.

Patients' contributions to the smooth running of the team?

Feedback

No human system can function without feedback. We cannot communicate effectively with anyone unless some sounds or gestures are returned. Similarly with health care. Unless we have some responses, we do not know how we are doing. We have a choice, either to do nothing and wait for feedback, or go out and seek it, so that we can get useful input into planning and running the service. Feedback can be negative, in the form of complaints; or it can be positive, in the form of constructive suggestions, often accompanied by offers of help. For example, when consulted about an information leaflet patients often produce good ideas, and they may know someone who will get it typeset and printed for next-to-nothing.

Health promotion and prevention of illness.

The success of attempts to prevent illness and promote health depend heavily on tuning in to the patient's health beliefs and perceptions of risk (King 1983). By involving patients in such programmes, their success is enhanced. This has a particular relevance for the achievement of screening targets and attempts to influence people's lifestyle. In one cervical screening programme, the uptake was doubled after a patient re-worded the letter of invitation.

Linking the team to community networks

Many of the determinants of health and illness lie outside the boundaries of medicine and health services, such as the presence of social support to people living alone, or families with multiple problems, poor housing and education. Much of the caring for the elderly disabled is by volunteers. Members of health care teams may need the help of key people in the community who are in touch with these services. In this way the health care team can achieve more effective action for the sort of problems that fall in the gaps between statutory services.

Forming a 'patient advisory group'

General practices that have patient groups find them very helpful, and the initial images (or nightmares) of the GPs being manipulated by their 'heart-sink' patients are soon dispelled. Patients are so delighted to be asked to help—in effect to join the team—that they usually respond positively. Getting a patient group started and keeping it going are not easy tasks, and require good management and communication skills. But once firmly established, patients contribute skills, energy and resources to do whatever they think is worthwhile. Instead of raising the GPs' anxieties, such a group goes a long way to allaying them. Ideas, fears for the future and plans can be discussed and the problems shared.

If team members (in general practice or hospital) wish to pursue the idea, what could they do about it? The first step might be for one member of the team to find out about patient groups, by visiting a local one, reading about them, and perhaps inviting someone from a similar group to attend a meeting. A 'start up booklet' can be obtained from the Royal College of General Practitioners (Pritchard 1993). Professionals, not only GPs, have worries about 'stirring up a hornet's nest'. These fears are natural and are based on the tradition of professional secrecy, which was thought, at one time, to be necessary for professional survival. Times have changed, and we are living in an age of freedom of information and participation, but professional attitudes do not change so quickly, as is indicated by the small number of such groups (about 3 per cent of UK practices, but increasing). For this team-building project, something short of a full patient advisory group is suggested.

Learning exercise 10: Patient participation

In this exercise we discuss ways that patients can be involved in helping the team with its preventive and curative work, ways that the team can come to see things more from the patient's viewpoint, and starting a dialogue with patients for the improvement of services. We also develop action plans for involving patients in teamwork.

Aim: To consider increased patient involvement in the
                   work of the team.

Objectives: By the end of the session participants will have:

(1) read the relevant recommended reading and collated suggestions from patients on
(a) the preventative, and
(b) the curative aspects of the service provided;

(2) compared lists previously compiled;

(3) discussed ways in which the team might respond to the
suggestions;

(4) discussed the ways in which patients might help the team to
function more effectively;

(5) produced an action plan based on discussion in (3) and (4);

(6) **Optional**—explored how patient involvement can be expanded.

Each team member has been asked to read Section 10 (pp.
99–101), and bring to the meeting two cards listing suggestions
from patients, one card about curative services and one about
prevention.

If necessary, allow 5 minutes to read Section 10. Working in
groups of two to four (from different disciplines), compare the
lists you have made. Discuss ways in which the team might
respond to the suggestions from patients, and ways in which
patients might help the team to function more effectively.

Re-form the main group to compare the results of the group
discussions, and make action plans, to be carried out as a sub-
project.

How could patients' ideas and suggestions be sought and acted
upon in the future? What other patient links or dialogues might
help?

Facilitator summary

Materials: *Lists of patients' suggestions*

Activity: *Ask participants to split into multidisciplinary sets and compare lists made.*

Encourage discussion of (i) Team response to patient suggestions, (ii) Ways patients might help the team function more effectively (15 min).

Re-form main group. Compare results of small group discussions. Formulate action plans based on these (40 min).

Optional *(extra time needed). Ask:*
(i) What further plans could be made?
(ii) How could patients' ideas and suggestions be acted on in future?
(iii) What other patient links and dialogues might help?

For the next meeting

Please read Section 11 (pp. 107–13) about evaluating the effectiveness of the team. Complete the pro forma (see next page), and bring it, unsigned, to the meeting as a basis for discussion. It will be collected and used as material for planning the way forward in Section 12 and subsequently.

QUESTIONNAIRE ON EVALUATION OF TEAMWORK

1. Achieving goals

List three key goals (refer back to Section 3) and ring the number which best represents the extent to which you feel that progress has been made towards their achievement.

	None					*Fully*
Goal 1	0	1	2	3	4	5
Goal 2	0	1	2	3	4	5
Goal 3	0	1	2	3	4	5

What will you be able to see, hear or feel that will tell you that each goal has been achieved? *Describe the evidence* you will have of achievement of the goal.

Goal 1 ....

Goal 2 ....

Goal 3 ....

Comments ....

....

2. Changes in the quality of teamwork since starting the project

Since the project started, I think the following changes have occurred (mark X in one column for each item:

	Much worse	Worse	Same	Better	Much better
A. Clear definition of goals					
B. Clear definition of roles					
C. Use of effective procedures					
D. Quality of interpersonal relationships					

Comments ....

....

....

3. Measuring and charting the benefits of teamwork

(a) Describe what you think is the best single measure of effective teamwork for your own team.

....

....

....

(b) How can you monitor, in terms that you can see, hear or feel, whether this measure is increasing or reducing?

....

....

(c) In relation to the measure you have just described, what action can you take to increase it, and to chart the increase?

....

....

Comments ....

....

Please bring completed questionnaires to the next meeting, for collection after the meeting.

E Evaluation of teamwork and the way forward

Section 11: Evaluating the effectiveness of the team

Why evaluate?

Evaluation is an essential ingredient of the management of any activity. This important statement has been made already in this book. Yet evaluation of team effectiveness is a neglected subject. Unless we discover whether we have achieved our aims, we will be lost. We will not know if all our efforts have been wasted, nor will we know if any changes we have made have improved or worsened patient care. We will have little idea of the best route to take next.

However, we need not be put off evaluating teamwork because there are no easy measures. All the members of the team are skilled evaluators of clinical or social states. They can apply this skill to the state of health of the team—to take its temperature and pulse and listen to its heartbeat—and apply their judgement to their observations and feelings.

Any professional who serves the public has duties prescribed, often by law such as a duty of care, or to keep records, or to write certificates. They also enjoy privileges, such as high public esteem and the freedom to take everyday decisions without referring to anyone else. This 'professional autonomy' is a valuable prize, but it has to be earned. Professional freedom must be matched by professional accountability (Pritchard 1986) if we are to retain public confidence and continue as a self-regulating profession. It is in everyone's interest that people working in health care give an account of their stewardship to those who have a legitimate stake in the quality of care and the service they provide. This is referred to as quality assurance (or quality improvement or quality management), and the means to provide it is audit, both of technical care and of the functioning of the organization.

Who needs us to evaluate—who are the stakeholders?

Ourselves

An essential part of professional identity and self-esteem is the feeling that we are doing a good job. Do we take this for granted, or do we try to find out if our standards do actually measure up to those of our peers? This topic of 'self-audit' is beyond the scope of this book.

Our professional peers

In order to hold their heads high, professionals must earn the respect of their peers. In the context of health care teams, this extends to professionals in all disciplines. A major message of this book has been the need to know about and value the work of colleagues in other disciplines. By 'sharing responsibility for outcome' we become stakeholders in each other's activity.

Health authorities and other statutory bodies

Nearly all health professionals work under contract with authorities or trusts who need to ensure that work is done up to standard and public money is well spent. They cannot directly intervene in the confidential work of the professional, but they need to be convinced that some sort of audit or quality assurance is operating.

Patients

Accountability to patients should be high on the list, but in a publicly funded service this may not be so. They, more than anyone, have a stake in the evaluation of the quality of their own health and health care.

The population served by the team

More and more we are trying to find out ways of determining need, so that we can serve all the population equitably. This underlies the enhanced importance of teamwork for implementing the recommendations of The Health of the Nation report (DoH 1992). Without effective teamwork, little will be achieved. Priorities have to be established between demand and need and between prevention and cure. Without measures this is reduced to guess-work.

Society at large

Conflict between the interests of 'society' and the individual or the local population is an everyday experience. Team members may have to make very difficult decisions when these conflicts arise. Yet we cannot operate in limbo, but only as a part of the larger group of human-kind.

How can we come to terms with being pulled in six directions? Fortunately most of the stakeholders want the same thing, but not always. We can only survive by reconciling the various interests when they differ, and putting ourselves in a position where our judgement is trusted by the stakeholders. This is more likely to happen when we are seen to be evaluating our work whenever possible.

What can we evaluate?

In order to evaluate we must measure, hence the earlier insistence on having measurable goals. Some measures may be precise and objective, like births, deaths or positive laboratory tests. Some may be subjective, like patient satisfaction, but this should not belittle it, as it is one of the most important outcome measures of health care. We need to evaluate the quality of team care using measures that are carefully selected, in order to help us achieve our goals.

We may concentrate on measures of specific risk factors such as levels of blood pressure, obesity, or smoking in the population, on the lines of the successful 'Rent an Audit' (Gray *et al.* 1987); we may evaluate clinical treatment such as in asthma or diabetes; or we may try to evaluate the effectiveness of the organization, for example the team. The advantage of the last approach is that an effective team is a 'multipurpose tool' which should serve us well in many areas of our work.

Evaluating teamwork—measures available

At the start of the book we described team structures that might be considered effective, for example intrinsic and functional teams. The 'team diagnostic instrument' was used earlier in the project. This gave us a good idea of the ways in which team processes operated. If the processes operate well there is a chance of a good outcome for the patient and for the team. One thing is certain—bad processes rarely produce good outcomes.

Outcome is what really matters, but outcome measures are hard to find in health care teamwork. This does not mean that we should not try to find them, but we may have to settle for process measures—measures of what we actually do. Fortunately, some process measures, like immunization, controlling high blood pressure or following guidelines, are closely linked to outcome, and are described as intermediate outcomes. We know that immunization against diphtheria is effective, so from measuring the process of immunization we can predict outcome.

Measures of team performance are not well developed, and there is scope for teams to develop their own. For example, we can look at our team goals developed in Section 3, and see how we can measure their achievement. This will be considered in the practical exercise.

Poulton and West (1993) have described a pluralistic approach to measuring the quality of teamwork. Their criteria include:

- the views and judgement of people concerned, such as patients, staff, authorities, other professional teams, using appropriate criteria;
- the innovativeness of the team;
- team vision and shared objectives;
- 'participative safety', implying that the team is seen by members as supportive and that information is safe within the team;
- commitment to excellence—a shared concern for quality of team and individual performance.

This is an ambitious attempt to research some yardsticks of team effectiveness which is long overdue. Meanwhile, we must use more pedestrian criteria. Procedures (considered in Section 5) can be evaluated. For example, does an examination of the message book reveal that some messages are not acknowledged or not acted upon. A study of the minutes of meetings may reveal that some decisions have not been implemented and some target dates have slipped by unnoticed. What are the time intervals between the first message about a stroke patient at home and the services and nursing aids being in place? How often are callers unable to telephone team members because the line is constantly engaged?

Computer-assisted evaluation

Collecting data for evaluation is hard work. With an efficient computer system, certain data can be monitored automatically. For example, Lawrence, Coulter, and Jones (1990) described a computerized audit of preventive procedures in 45 practices. In this way, each team could see how they were doing in relation to other members of the group. They found that good performance correlated with smaller lists and more ancillary staff being available. There is no doubt that imaginative use of conventional practice computer systems will allow more effective evaluation to be done at less cost in time, energy, and money. But the team members would still need to look at the data, take decisions, implement action plans, and evaluate their effectiveness.

There are strong arguments for audit data from different units to be comparable, but teams would be well advised to do their own data collection and analysis, where possible. In this way the information will be relevant for clinical decisions and for management of the team, as well as a part of the wider information strategy.

Benefits of teamwork

In Section 1 (p. 16) some possible advantages of teamwork were listed. Can we find any evidence to support these statements, and if so what evidence? For example:

1. Can we show that teamwork benefits continuity of care? If so, how would we measure it?

2. Do patients prefer teamwork, and how can we show that is true?

3. Is teamwork a more efficient way of getting things done, and is this measurable?

4. Can we show that our capacity for learning from each other is enhanced?

5. Is job satisfaction at an acceptable level? Is it rising or falling?

6. As a result of teamwork, are preventive and curative services better integrated? Can we find some measurable examples?

We are often too eager to find fault with ourselves and others. The team will build confidence more rapidly if emphasis is put on success, with due celebration of our achievements.

Costs of teamwork

Teamwork uses up members' time and energy. Its cash cost is minimal. But could the time and energy be better used? How can we measure these as net costs, bearing in mind that teamwork may use time, but can also save time?

Though team members should have ways of avoiding or re-solving conflict, there is always the risk that by getting closer to one another at work any contradictions in values or beliefs will be highlighted, with conflict as a consequence. If this shows signs of becoming destructive of our daily work, then help should be sought, as outlined in Section 8.

Empathic teamwork

Teamwork also exacts a toll at a more emotional level. For pro-fessionals to look critically at their role, in terms of how members of other disciplines see them, is not easy. Likewise, to try to understand the viewpoints and roles of other team members requires an effort of will. Without this humble approach, and a commitment to 'get into each other's shoes', teams are less likely to work well. Yet health professionals spend much of their time with patients doing exactly that, and call it empathizing. Applying to the team process the skills that work with patients, can pay off in better teamwork, based on closer understanding and sympathy.

Learning exercise 11: Evaluating teamwork

In this exercise we evaluate teamwork in terms of achieving key goals, changes in the quality of teamwork since starting the project, and selecting one measure of effective teamwork for further study.

Aim: To evaluate teamwork in terms of achieving key goals, and of the measurement of change in the quality of teamwork since the beginning of this project.

Objectives: By the end of the session participants will have:

(1) read the recommended reading and completed the questionnaires;

(2) discussed the questionnaire results;

(3) collated and summarized the results of the questionnaires.

Members have been asked to complete questionnaires about achieving key goals, changes in the quality of teamwork, and ways of measuring and charting the benefits of teamwork. If necessary, allow 5 minutes to read Section 12. Working in groups of two to four, discuss the completed questionnaires. Allow 10 minutes for each section (30 minutes).

Re-form the main group to allow a member of each group in turn to give a brief report on their results. Select one or two 'measures of effective teamwork' and make action plans to monitor them as a sub-project.

The questionnaire responses should be collected for collation, and the summarized results given to the team members before the next meeting.

Facilitator summary

Materials: *Completed questionnaires.*

Activity: *Revision of recommended reading (5 min).*

Ask participants to split into multidisciplinary sets to discuss the completed questionnaires (30 min). Allow 10 minutes for each section.

Re-form main group. Ask for results from each group.

Select one or two measures of effective teamwork, as agreed by the group, to make action plans for monitoring them. (Collate the questionnaire responses to give summarized results at the next session.) (25 min).

For the next meeting

Please read Section 12, and plan to talk about any sub-projects you are responsible for. Also, bring for discussion and review any action plans that have been made.

Section 12: The way forward

At the end of a review period, in the case of this project of 13 weekly sessions, we can take stock of how far we are along the road we wish to take and what our future goals and routes will be. We may now find that we have a very different picture of our future. This is part of the so-called 'management cycle' which is really a spiral, as it does not end up where it started. Teamwork and team development are an integral and important part of the management process as a whole. In this session we suggest that participants try to build a bridge, whereby the results and ideas from the team development project can rejoin the continuing management process. For this reason, the questionnaire for Section 11 (pp. 104–6) has been long and searching, and material from other sessions can be considered too, particularly concerning goals. This might be an appropriate moment to ask a number of questions, for example:

1. What are our key goals now?

2. Have we begun to achieve the goals we formulated earlier?

3. What is the 'state of health' of our team?

4. What do we plan to do to keep it (or make it) healthy?

5. What sub-projects have we started, and what progress are they making?

6. Have we identified further development or training needs? What action do we propose to take about them?

These questions will indicate that the end of the planned team development project is, in reality, just a marker along the route of continuing personal and team development. The project may have equipped team members with a tool kit or vehicle to make the journey into the future easier and more rewarding. The ultimate aim is for health care to become more effective in meeting the health needs of the population that the team aims to serve, and also to ensure that it is a fulfilling activity for all the staff, both professional and lay, who participate in it.

Learning exercise 12: Assessing progress

In this exercise we assess progress so far on the basis of the data collected during the project and the evaluative data from the previous session, and address issues for the future in terms of overall management, of further team development and further education.

Aim: To assess progress so far and make necessary plans for the future based on this assessment.

Objectives: At the end of the session participants will have:

1. read the recommended reading;

2. read through previous sub-project plans;

3. assessed progress on previous projects;

4. listed action necessary for future plans.

In the main group, spend about 5 minutes on reviewing each of the sub-projects (refer back to summary Fig. 1 in the Introduction, p. 7), then consider:

- How are we doing as a team?

- Where do we go from here?

- Have we made and agreed action plans, with target dates for completion and evaluation?

- Have we agreed who should be responsible for each action plan?

A review of progress to date and plans for future action should follow.

Facilitator summary

Materials: *Note from previous sub-projects.*

Activity: *Review of any sub-projects undertaken (10 min) (shown as **optional** on previous notes).*

Encourage team to discuss:

(i) How they are now as a team,

(ii) Where do they want to go from here (50 min).

Make an action plan for further development.

F Building effective shared care

Section 13: Tools for shared care

Some current trends

The general practitioner, in most European countries, remains a generalist against a background of increasing medical specialization, and may be a gatekeeper to non-emergency hospital care. The general practitioner has to hold the balance and refer appropriately. This is no easy task, as reflected in widely different referral rates and conflict about what problems should be referred (Hopkins and Wallace 1992; Roland and Coulter 1992).

Shared, or integrated, care assumes greater importance as ideas change and resources come under closer scrutiny. Shared care, whereby responsibility is divided between the primary care team and the specialist team, aims to allow the patient to spend more time, and receive a higher quality of care outside the hospital. Telemedicine, whereby the problem can be referred for specialist opinion, not the patient, should increase this trend.

General practitioner fundholding in Britain tends to focus on episodes of hospital care that can be costed, such as cold surgery, rather than on the continuing care of chronic illness and disability and the needs of the elderly. This runs counter to the British Government commitment to 'The Health of the Nation' priorities, which mirror those of the World Health Organization. These priorities should reinforce the importance of shared care in order to improve the effectiveness and equity of services as well as giving value for money.

What is shared care?

The term shared care applies when:

The responsibility for care of the patient is shared between individuals or teams which are part of separate organizations.

This definition makes the distinction between teamwork, where people work closely together with common goals and tasks, and shared care which, in organizational terms, is even more complex than teamwork.

Shared care is complex largely by reason of numbers. For teams to work effectively, they have to be small (say ten people) and preferably work under the same roof. General practitioners and specialists rarely work under the same roof[1], and the numbers involved can be large. For example in a Health District with a population of 250 000 served by a district general hospital, there are likely to be at least 20 specialist teams interested in shared care (out of a total of 56 recognized specialist categories). About 125 general practitioners arranged in 30 practice teams would serve the population. The number of links between teams would be 600. The number of individuals involved would be around 500.

The conclusion is clear. Cooperation as a team, with shared vision, goals, and procedures, is out of reach. There would be no time left to do the job. Short cuts and an effective system of cooperation are needed.

Every domain is different

There are 56 registered specialties in Britain, and communication and cooperation across the boundary with primary and community services is essential. Shared care is particularly important when the hospital supplies technology or services not available to the primary health care team (such as obstetrics or renal dialysis). Regular surveillance has not been a tradition in general practice, but this is changing, for example in the care of diabetes. Other domains where shared care is common are palliative care, mental illness, the elderly, rheumatic disorders, asthma, cardiovascular disease, and many more. Each of these domains has a very different structure and requirements, and each must be planned and developed to suit local circumstances. No overall blueprint is possible, but some common methodology—some tools for shared care—can be sought.

Developing shared care

Cooperation between teams working at different sites, in different organizations, and with different goals and methods is a difficult undertaking. Yet examples of successful shared care have shown that it can work well in improving outcomes in certain domains such as diabetes and obstetrics. Seven steps to effective shared care are outlined below.

1. Develop effective teamwork in all teams

As a first step, each team needs to put its own house in order by ensuring that they are indeed a team, with shared goals, and understanding of each other's roles, effective procedures, and adequate interpersonal relationships. A good start to shared care might be to work through this book. If team function is satisfactory, team members will have the ability and confidence to build cooperative relationships with other teams, as described below. If the team is dysfunctional, this will adversely affect professional work as well as morale.

2. Develop a shared understanding of the domain

Unless all concerned in shared care have a common understanding of, for example, the nature and treatment of diabetes and its complications, they will have different expectations and their common purpose will disintegrate. One way of developing this common understanding, which has worked well in the care of diabetes in Sweden (Carlson 1990), is to use 'conceptual modelling'. This is a technical term for getting ideas out in the open. The initial session involves patients, specialists, general practitioners, nurses, social workers, and other staff involved in the domain. They hold a brainstorming session in which named objects are written on cards and stuck on the wall. All the cards are then linked by lines to which a verb is added. In this way, everyone can share their perceptions and come to a common understanding of the disease and what it is like to suffer from it. From that beginning, goal and flow models are constructed and agreed, and an action plan developed.

The conceptual modelling session is best coordinated by a facilitator, such as a diabetes specialist nurse, who could then carry on with the process in other teams throughout the district, so that each primary health care team can jointly develop its own organization and plan.

3. Develop and implement guidelines

The action plan inevitably leads to agreed procedures and guidelines (protocols). By involving all those concerned, including patients, in the development of the procedures and guidelines, they have a better chance of success. Initiating guidelines needs extensive research into all reliable data on the topic. This is a major task, best undertaken by a national institute but implemented locally. The work will be made easier when the Cochrane Collaboration bears fruit (Chalmers *et al.* 1992), and all validated data can be accessed electronically. This will produce a world database of written knowledge, which is a good starting point. Firm evidence is accruing of the effectiveness of guidelines in changing general practitioners behaviour (Russell and Grimshaw 1993).

Guidelines will be needed in all the domains of shared care, and many other aspects of the general practitioner's work, such as diagnosis, investigation, prescribing, preventive and anticipatory care, and referral. This is likely to total several hundred guidelines. For these to be held on paper and accessed manually is unrealistic. An early task must be to get all guidelines on to the computer, so that they can be accessed instantly during the consultation. Unless they can be integrated and employed in a flexible manner, they are unlikely to be valued by the doctor, and will fall into disuse.

4. Develop effective communication and learning

The facilitator has a key role in the knowledge transfer and developing links and procedures between all the parties to co-operation. New technology is a trigger for change and also provides a medium for learning. Management of change is a key to success, and teams need to function as 'learning organizations' (AMED 1993; Senge 1992; Swieringa and Wierdsma 1992). Key features of a learning organization are listed below:

- A team must be driven by their vision of the future, not the past, (though they can learn from the past).
- The values and the priorities of the team, and of team members, must be made explicit. Values cannot all be shared, but they need to be understood and accepted.
- All team members must be open and prepared to innovate and to acknowledge mistakes made and lessons learned.
- Learning needs to be combined with doing in all the team's activities. Improvement in learning must be acknowledged and rewarded, not just improvement in performance.
- Team strategies and plans should be flexible. Planning must be seen as a learning process (for example care plans).
- Information appropriate for carrying out tasks must be shared openly, and updated in response to learning by experience.
- Training must be a catalyst for further learning and doing.
- Becoming a learning organization is a fundamental change, and must be managed as such.

(Modified from Pritchard, W. (1992). Notes on the learning organization (personal communication).)

5. Implement decision support

People do not have just one diagnosis, and there are numerous determinants of illness; namely, medical, social, and psychological. Patients have preferences which need to be taken into account, so numerous alternative pathways for shared care need to be considered. Alternatives need to be made explicit, so that the doctor's judgement can be brought into play, rather than jumping to a 'best fit'. All these factors demonstrate the limited role that conventional computer systems can play in this very complex field. Implementation of decision support for shared care has the advantage that priority domains can be selected first, and a modular development path followed. This presupposes a comprehensive system, such as the Oxford System of Medicine (Fox *et al.* 1990, Gordon 1991), so that the modules can eventually be integrated. Development of decision support is well advanced, and should be available in two or three years time.

6. Implement evaluation of processes and outcomes

Clinical audit consumes the time and energy of clinicians in checking what they are convinced are sound decisions and favourable outcomes. Only the very energetic and dedicated pursue it as a continuing process of quality development on a broad front—not just their favourite diseases. It is no surprise that clinical audit has made so little progress. Yet in a climate of cost containment, it is all the more essential to ensure that patients get value for money, not just the cheapest option. Automatic audit using conventional computers has made progress, but the potential of knowledge-based systems for auditing outcomes still needs to be realized.

7. Link audit data with decision processes and guidelines

Conformity to guidelines in a knowledge-based system can be monitored before the decision is finally made, so providing 'concurrent audit' (Pritchard 1991). The potential for improving the quality of care is so great, that the cost of the system could be recouped in a very short time.

Once the automatic audit of outcomes is in place, it could be used as a (retrospective) audit of the decision processes and the guidelines. This would add a new dimension to medicine, in validating or refuting much of current clinical medical practice. Eventually, general practice would be able to develop a comprehensive knowledge base that reflected the prevalence of illness in primary health care.

The seven steps to developing shared care, now and in the future, are summarized in Table 1 below:

Section 14: The role and training of the facilitator

Throughout this workbook, the role of the facilitator has been stressed. Who are facilitators, and what role do they play in primary and shared care? What are their training needs and are these being filled? Some facilitators are employed to operate in primary care, some in secondary, and some in both.

The primary care facilitator

Over 300 facilitators are deployed in primary health care to assist with many functions, some of which are listed below:

- health promotion and prevention of illness;
- primary health care and service development;
- nurse training;
- quality of care development;
- team-building;
- diabetes, asthma, cardiovascular disease, mental health;
- ethnic minority issues;
- computerization.

The roles are diverse and training for them a major challenge (Allsop 1990). The National Facilitator Development Project has run a number of induction and refresher courses for facilitators. They have a new handbook for facilitators (Wilson 1994).

Table 1. Developing shared care—seven steps

Goals	Method	Key workers	Incentives
1. Well-functioning PHC and hospital teams	Team building exercise and continuing evaluation	Visionary leader Facilitator	Linked to resource allocation?
2. Develop a shared understanding of the domain and its organization	Conceptual modelling leading to organization design	Facilitator	Linked to resource allocation?
3. Develop shared guidelines/protocols	National guideline program. Adapt locally. Patient input	National Institute. Local domain enthusiasts. Facilitator	Central and local funding
4. Develop effective communication and learning	Shared record. Telemedicine. Smart card. 'Learning organization'	Local enthusiast. Facilitator.	Funding. External audit
5. Implement decision support	Involve users. Work on climate for change	Product champion. Teachers	Peer influence. Indemnity insurers
6. Evaluate and audit processes and outcomes	Concurrent and retrospective audit. Feedback to users.	Audit facilitator. Data clerk	Peer influence. Contract. Job satisfaction
7. Refine knowledge base and guidelines	Feedback of data into decision support system	User group. Expert editorial team	Validate medical knowledge and practice

A recent pilot training course was based on the strategy of developing a learning organization, with facilitators as change agents. A learning organization is one that is continually expanding its capacity to create its future, that is not just learning to adapt to the changing environment but learning in a way that enhances our capacity to create (Senge 1992).

The programme for this four-day interactive course was based on the results of a questionnaire sent to all primary care facilitators in 1992. From over 100 responses the key topics identified were:

- managing change;
- building effective teams;
- developing facilitative skills;
- linking primary health care to other organizations.

Facilitators need independence from the organizations they are trying to help. They should be both **structurally** independent (not subordinate in the organisation) and **psychologically** independent (not isolated from or colluding with the organization). Even if well set up structurally, there will come a point when the facilitator feels their psychological independence is threatened. This was borne out by the issues brought by the group of experienced facilitators who participated in a pilot course. Typical examples were:

'I have too many demands and find myself sucked in to the FHSA's needs.'

'The client may see me as a threat.'

'I am unsure whether I am giving too much or too little guidance.'

'I feel I don't know enough or have the skills to cope.'

These and other issues were used to design the content of the pilot course. The learning organization theme is approached on a number of different levels:

1. Models and case histories are discussed in the large group to increase theoretical understanding and provide insight into organizational processes.

2. Participants are engaged in the process of creating a learning organization in the group. Course tutors use issues that participants have brought to design the programme 'live' in front of the group.

3. In the small groups, specific obstacles are tackled which get in the way of the individuals' development and ability to help the organization to learn.

Some of the things participants found particularly helpful were:

'the developing nature of the course'

'the way expressed needs were used to inform and guide the group work'

'identifying roles and the ability to adapt learning to the individual needs'

'planning the programme around needs identified by the course participants'

Back at work, what did they do differently?

'felt more confident, clear, working better. Understand the issues better.'

'being more supportive and understanding to colleagues.'

'It's more subtle than "doing"—it's a change of thinking.'

The nature of the facilitator's work is that they can never know enough to feel fully competent in all situations. The aim of this course was for participants to get a sense of their own skills and resources for working in this difficult area. This comes from the new knowledge they acquire, new insights into the nature of facilitation, and a clearer understanding of what they bring to the job.

Facilitators in secondary and shared care

Facilitators based on secondary care are mostly based in hospital departments, but some may operate almost entirely in the community. They are a diverse group according to the domain, including hospice nurses, community psychiatric nurses, stoma nurses, and a host of others. Their importance is increasing with the implementation of care in the community.

Their role includes liaison, teaching, influencing, and negotiating. They may act as a patient's advocate, a researcher, an innovator, a counsellor, and a manager. The emphasis is on encouraging self-reliance and self-care by the patient, not fostering dependency.

In many cases they have a service role, and if this is undertaken in isolation from primary and community staff, the effect may be to deny them the opportunity to learn, and result in their leaving the work to the 'expert'. This may bring short-term technical benefit, but ends up de-skilling and demotivating the local staff. Hospital outposts and 'hospital at home' may be advantageous in certain circumstances, but the learning consequences have to be borne in mind.

Training of shared care facilitators

Training programmes vary according to the specialty and are not considered in detail here. Common training in shared skills, such as teaching, facilitating, bringing about change and teambuilding might be to everyone's advantage. The training needs arising from the Table 1—'Seven steps to shared care'—are as formidable as are the problems of implementing effective shared care.

References and further reading

Allsop, J. (1990). *Changing primary care. The role of facilitators.* The King's Fund, London.

AMED (1993). *Learning more about learning organizations.* AMED focus paper October 1993. Association for Management Education and Development, 21 Catherine Street, London WC2B 5JS. (£13 post free.)

Belbin, R. M. (1981). *Management teams: why they succeed or fail.* Heinemann, Oxford.

Byrne, P. S. and Long, B. E. (1976). *Doctors talking to patients: a study of the verbal behaviour of general practitioners consulting in their surgeries.* Department of Health and Social Security, HMSO, London. (Republished 1984 by Royal College of General Practitioners.)

Carlson, A. (1990). *Reforming diabetes care in general practice. Evaluation of two strategies for the development of the organisation and quality of health care.* Karolinska Institute, Stockholm University, Stockholm.

Chalmers, I. *et al.* (1992). Getting to grips with Archie Cochrane's agenda. All randomised controlled trials should be registered and reported. *British Medical Journal,* **305**, 786–8.

Clare, A. W. and Corney, R. H. (1982). *Social work and primary health care.* Academic Press, London.

DHSS. (1981). *The Primary health care team.* Report of a joint working group of the Standing Medical Advisory Committee and the Standing Nursing and Midwifery Advisory Committee. Department of Health, London. (Harding-Frost Report.)

DoH. (1992). The Health of the Nation. *A strategy for health in England.* HMSO, London. Cmd 1986.

Ellis, N. (1984). Looking after your new employee. *British Medical Journal,* **289**, 417–18.

Ellis, N. (1990). *Employing staff* (4th edn). British Medical Journal, London.

Fox, J. *et al.* (1990). Logic engineering for knowledge engineering: design and implementation of the Oxford System of Medicine. *Artificial Intelligence in Medicine*, **2**, 323–29.

Gilmore, M., Bruce, N., and Hunt, M. (1974). *The work of the nursing team in general practice.* Council for the Education and Training of Health Visitors, London.

Gordon C. (1991) Supporting acts. Primary care decision support. *British Journal of Healthcare Computing*, 29–30.

Hopkins, A. and Wallace, P. (ed.) (1992). *Referral to medical outpatients.* Royal College of Physicians, London.

Huntington, J. (1981a). *Social work and general medical practice: collaboration or conflict.* George Allen and Unwin, London.

Huntington, J. (1981b). Time orientations in the collaboration of social workers and general practitioners. *Social Science Medicine*, **15**A, 203.

Jones, R. V. H. (1986). *Working together: learning together.* Occasional Paper no: 33. Royal College of General Practitioners, London.

Jay, A. (1976). *How to run a meeting.* Booklet to accompany the film *Meetings, bloody meetings.* Video Arts, London.

King, J. (1983). Health beliefs in the consultation. In *Doctor–patient communication* (ed. D. Pendleton and J. Hasler), pp 109–25. Academic Press, London.

Lawrence, M. Coulter, A., and Jones, L. (1990). A total audit of preventive procedures in 45 practices caring for 430 000 patients. *British Medical Journal*, **300**, 1501–3.

Muir Gray, J. A. Muir *et al.* (1987). Rent-an-audit. *Journal of the Royal College of General Practioners* **37**, 177.

Pendleton, D. *et al.* (1984). *The consultation: an approach to learning and teaching.* Oxford University Press, Oxford.

Plovnick, M. S., Fry, R. E., and Rubin, I. R. (1978). *Managing health care delivery: a training program for primary care physicians.* Ballinger Publishing Company, Harvard, Mass.

Poulton, B. C. and West, M. A. (1993). Effective multidisciplinary teamwork in primary health care. *Journal of Advanced Nursing*, **18**, 918–25.

Pritchard, P. M. M. (1986). Professional accountability in general practice. In *The Medical Annual 1986* (ed. D. J. Pereira Gray and J. Pereira Gray), pp. 243–54. John Wright and Sons, Bristol.

Pritchard, P. M. M. (1981). *Manual of primary health care: its nature and organization* (2nd edn). Oxford University Press, Oxford.

Pritchard P. (1991). Can decision making be improved? *Postgraduate Education for General Practice*, **2**, 4–6.

Pritchard, P. M. M. (1992). Doctors, patients and time. In *Time and health* (ed. R. Frankenberg), pp. 75–93. Sage Publications, London.

Pritchard, P. M. M. (1993). *Partnership with patients. A practical guide to starting a patient participation group* (3rd edn). Royal College of General Practitioners, London.

Pritchard, P. M. M., Low, K., and Whalen, M. (1984). *Management in general practice*. Oxford University Press, Oxford.

Ratoff, L., Rose, A., and Smith, C. (1974). Social workers and GPs: problems of working together. *Social Work Today*, **5**, 497–500.

Revans, R. W. (1986). The origins and growth of action learning. In *Action learning in practice* (ed. M. Pedler) pp. 19–21. Gower Press, Aldershot.

Roland, M. and Coulter, A. (ed.) (1992). *Hospital referrals*. Oxford University Press, Oxford.

Rubin, I. R. and Beckhard, R. (1972). Factors influencing the effectiveness of health teams. *Milbank Memorial Fund Quarterly*, **5**, part 2, 317–35.

Rubin, I. R., Plovnick, M. S., and Fry, R. E. (1975). *Improving the coordination of care: a program for health team development*. Ballinger Publishing Company, Harvard, Mass.

Russell I. T. and Grimshaw, J. M. (1993). *The effectiveness of referral guidelines: a review of methods and findings of published evaluations*. In *Hospital referrals*, (ed. M. Roland and A. Coulter), pp. 179–211. Oxford University Press, Oxford.

Senge, P. E. (1992). *The Fifth Discipline. The art and practice of the learning organization*. Random House UK, London. (First published in USA in 1990.)

Swieringa, J. and Wierdsma, A. (1992). *Becoming a learning organization. Beyond the learning curve*. Addison-Wesley, Wokingham.

Vaill, P. B. (1982). The purposing of high-performing systems. *Organizational Dynamics*. Autumn 1982. AMACOM Periodicals Division, American Management Associations.

Wilson, A., (1994). *Changing practices in primary care. A facilitator's handbook*. Health Education Authority UK, London.

Useful addresses

CAIPE (Centre for Advancement of Inter-Professional Education) 344 Gray's Inn Road, London WC1X 8BP. Tel. 071 278 4411.

An organization that aims to stimulate education in inter-disciplinary teamwork in UK and Europe. Chairman: Dr John Horder.

HEA PHC Unit (Health Education Authority Primary Health Care Unit) Churchill Hospital, Headington, Oxford OX3 7LJ. Tel. 0865 60267 or 0865 226061, Fax. 0865 741980.

This unit has made a great impact on team development, by setting up workshops and networks nationwide. Producing a database of relevant references and resources, and a facilitators' manual.

The Industrial Society Peter Runge House, 3 Carlton House Terrace, London SW1Y 5DG. Tel. 071 839 4300.

Publishes useful booklets on topics such as motivation and use of time. Has regional offices.

King's Fund Centre 126 Albert Street, London NW1 7NF. Tel. 071 267 6111.

Carries out a number of activities in connection with primary health care development. Site of the Quality Improvement Project, and publisher of numerous booklets on quality assurance and PHC development. Excellent library on these topics.

King's Fund College 2 Palace Court, London W2 4HS. Tel. 071
727 0581.
   Management training college, and runs workshops on team
development.

National Facilitator Development Project Miss Elaine Fullard,
Project Director, Sue Lister Development Officer, Block 10,
The Churchill Hospital, Headington, Oxford OX3 7LJ. Tel. 0865
226052/3, Fax, 0865 741980.

Royal College of General Practitioners 14 Princes Gate,
London SW7 1PU.
   Information resources centre and library.

Video Arts Ltd Dumbarton House, 68 Oxford Street, London
W1N 9LA. Tel. 071 637 7288.
   Publishes booklets, and hires out films and videos on a
number of management topics. Particularly relevant to team
development are the *Unorganized manager* series; *Meetings,
bloody meetings* and its sequels; and a number of videos on
communication. These videos are very professionally produced,
and mostly star John Cleese. They have proved popular with
team members.

Freelance consultants
Dr June Huntington
23 Daleham Gardens
London NW3 5BY   Tel. 071 435 1356; Fax. 071 431 0377

Donald Mungall
Littlecroft
Portsmouth Road
Esher
Surrey KT10 9JB   Tel. 0372 64986; Fax. 0372 64738

James Pritchard Associates
3 Boults Close
Old Marston
Oxford OX3 0PP   Tel. 0865 241854; Fax. 0865 210844

Ms Nicki Spiegal
6 Boston Court
Brownhill Road
Chandlers Ford
Hampshire SO5 2EH   Tel. 0703 252323

Mrs Kathryn Wilkinson (née Evans)
37 Carlisle Avenue
St Albans
Herts AL3 5LX   Tel. 0727 56684

Field testing: Authors' note

This workbook has been field tested in a number of primary health care teams. The authors would like this process to be continuous, in order to improve the acceptability and effectiveness of this workbook. Members of any teams who have used the workbook are invited to send their ideas and suggestions to one of the authors (addresses below). A check-list used in the field testing follows. All contributions will be treated as confidential and acknowledged.

Peter Pritchard
31 Martin's Lane
Dorchester on Thames
Oxon OX10 7JF
(Tel 0865 340 008)
(Fax 0865 341 593)

James Pritchard
3 Boults Close
Old Marston
Oxford OX3 0PP
(Tel 0865 241 854)
(Fax 0865 240 844)

TEAMWORK FOR PRIMARY and SHARED CARE
Feedback check-list

1. Name of practice, department, or unit

2. Name of facilitator (if any), or contributor

3. Size of group (average)

4. Membership of group by job function (**not** names)

5. Was an external facilitator used—if so for which exercises?

6. Was the process carried out as suggested in the introduction?
   If not, how was it carried out? Any other comments on the way the book was used?

7. **For each section**, please answer the following?
   (a) numbers attending?
   (b) what went well, or was helpful to the team?
   (c) what did not go well, or was unhelpful?

   These comments could be written on the appropriate page of a master copy to be returned to the authors, or separate pro formas could be used for each section. In addition, please make any corrections or suggestions in the master copy, preferably in red.

8. If the practice agree, please attach a copy of the completed questionnaires from Section 11 (pp. 104–6), together with any conclusions from the discussion in Exercise 12 (p. 117), and general suggestions about improving the workbook.

   Would contributors (or facilitators) please return the evaluation results to the authors as soon as possible?

   With many thanks for your cooperation.

Index

T

WITHDRAWN
FROM STOCK
QMUL LIBRARY